Heal Yourself

Heal Yourself

The Secrets of Your Mind and Body

Ryuho Okawa

JAICO PUBLISHING HOUSE

Ahmedabad Bangalore Bhopal Chennai
Delhi Hyderabad Kolkata Lucknow Mumbai

Published by Jaico Publishing House
A-2 Jash Chambers, 7-A Sir Phirozshah Mehta Road
Fort, Mumbai - 400 001
jaicopub@jaicobooks.com
www.jaicobooks.com

First published as *'Kokoro-to-Karada-no-Honto-no-Kankei'*
by IRH Press Co., Ltd.

Published in arrangement with
IRH Press Co., Ltd.
Tokyo, Japan

To be sold only in India, Bangladesh, Bhutan,
Pakistan, Nepal, Sri Lanka and the Maldives.

HEAL YOURSELF
ISBN 978-81-8495-397-8

First Jaico Impression: 2013

Printed by
Trinity Academy For Corporate Training Limited, Mumbai

Contents

Chapter 2

The Spiritual Truth about Mind and Body

Part II

Q&A Effective Advice for Mind and Body

Chapter 1
Healing Your Mind

Chapter 2
About Various Diseases

Chapter 3
For Nurses and Caregivers

The Mind and the Physical Body

No one

Willingly longs to become ill.

Yet, large hospitals

Are as busy and crowded as supermarkets.

In truth, your subconsciousness is seeking illness,

Even though your consciousness might not be.

When you experience a setback at work,

When you are exhausted by your studies,

When you are reprimanded,

When you are humiliated and your dignity is hurt,
When you feel hesitant to ask for a vacation,
When you face feelings of inferiority or limitations
In your knowledge and skills,
When you feel like a hopeless failure,
When you are being crushed by the weight
Of people's massive expectations,
When there is no outlet for your stress,
When you become pessimistic,

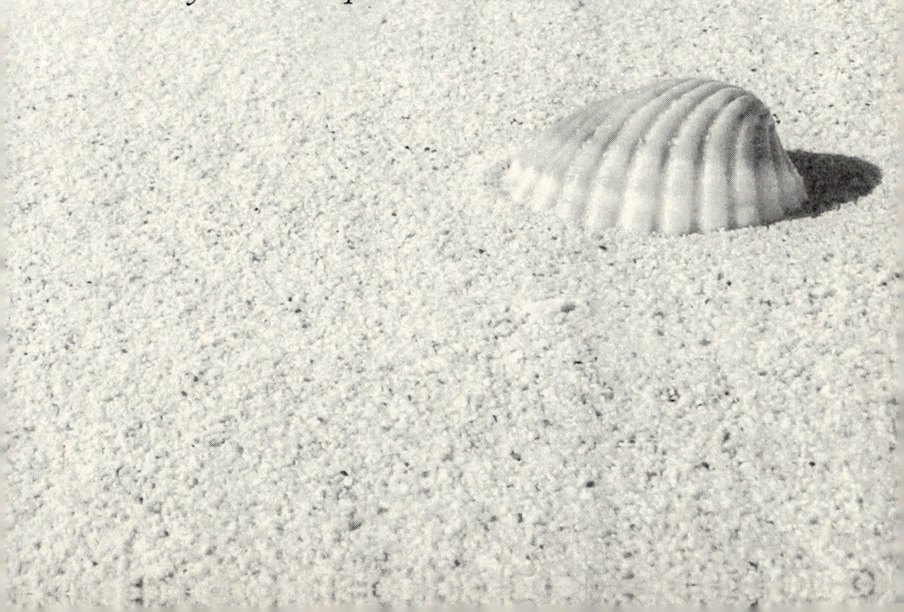

When you cannot improve your bad habits,
When you are plagued by a sense of guilt.

By now, I am sure you have realized,
That illnesses are formed when your mind weakens.
So pray, believe, and
Strengthen your will to recover.
Your body will respond to that will.
Believe that you are by nature, strong and healthy.

Hope,
Determination,
And Buddha's Truth,
Will dramatically increase
Your body's power to heal.

Ryuho Okawa
President of Happy Science

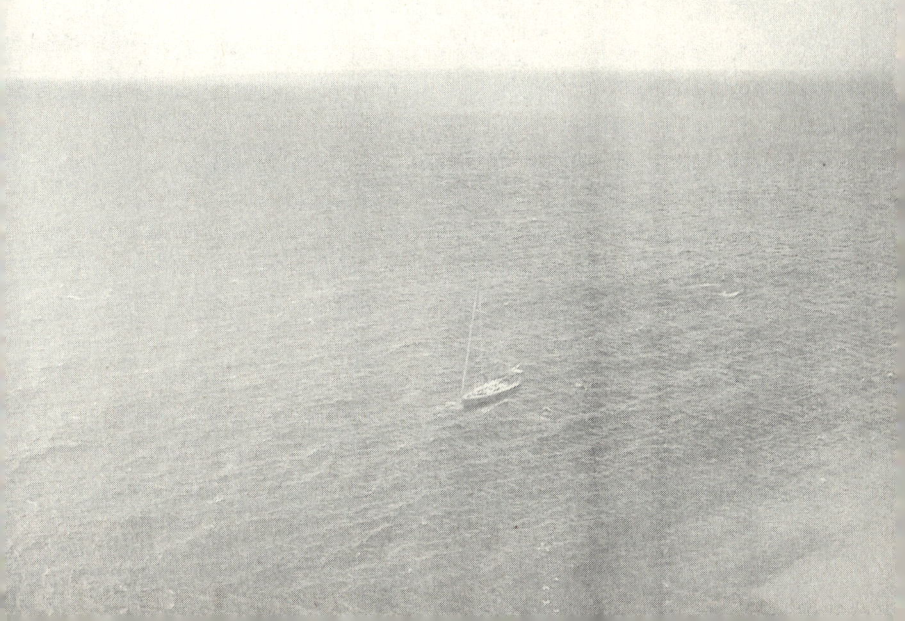

Part I

Building a Happy Relationship Between Mind and Body

Part I Chapter 1

How to Live a Healthy Lifestyle

1

Surviving Our Stressful Modern Society

A healthy lifestyle is extremely important, a treasure that money cannot buy. Having good control of the body and maintaining a healthy lifestyle are the keys to living happily for a long time. This will allow you to enjoy your life without inconveniencing others.

In most cases, people who become sick have been overdoing things, or they have become too careless. Likewise, injuries mostly occur because the injured person was not paying attention. Those who concentrate on the spiritual aspect of things sometimes are prone to think lightly about the body. However, without a healthy body it is difficult to enjoy a sustained feeling of happiness.

You have to bear in mind that the body and spirit are interrelated. In the other world, we only have our mind but in this world the body and mind influence each other. Thus, if the mind is sick, then the body will also become ill. Conversely, if the body is sick, the state of mind too will become worse.

Today, the number of people dying from cancer is on the rise, and actually, in nearly all cases the root cause is spiritual stress, anxiety or anguish.

People's minds materialize. That is why the state of the mind immediately affects the body, and the physical condition undergoes change. If the mind becomes ill, then the body will begin to suffer too.

I am not saying that "bad people get cancer." In a stressful society like ours, controlling one's mind is difficult, and without even knowing it we end up continuously pushing ourselves too far. So in many cases this pressure, including spiritual exhaustion, terror, needless worrying about the future and general misgivings, causes people to become ill.

If your spiritual condition deteriorates, the body will

begin to reflect it. There are many cases in which people have fallen physically ill because their company had gone bankrupt and deep into debt. In such instances, the mind gives up before the body does.

Furthermore, if the body becomes ill, the spirit too will steadily rot away, resulting in more and more discontent and complaints. You might end up saying sharp words to other people and venting your anger indiscriminately on them, leading to disharmony with those around you. In short, if the body is ill, the mind too, will become ill.

Consequently, we must realize that, as Buddhism puts it: "In this world, the body and mind are united and cannot be divided—they influence one another." Therefore, the care of the body is extremely important.

Proper nutrition, the right amount of exercise and the appropriate degree of rest—these are the keys to health. You have to pay attention to nutrition, commit yourself to exercise, and make sure that you are getting enough sleep. Balance among the trio of nutrition, exercise and rest creates a healthy lifestyle. It is that simple. If your physical condition becomes poor, this three-pronged balance has been destroyed; therefore, you must be mindful of maintaining this balance.

2

Mind is to Body as Driver is to Car

Children receive a genetic blueprint from their parents, and their body develops in line with this schematic design. However, the influence of environmental factors is more than half responsible for what kind of body will ultimately develop.

For example, even if the parents were athletes who have robust physiques, if their children did not engage in sports, they will not develop the same kind of physiques that their parents had. Moreover, even if the parents are bright intellectuals, if their children do not sufficiently devote themselves to their studies, then they will not follow the examples of their mother and father. Even if there is a blueprint to a certain extent, how things will eventually turn out will vary widely between individuals.

Here we can make a comparison to the relationship between a car and its driver, with the body being the car and the soul being the driver. Two different drivers will drive the same exact car in vastly different ways. If the person knows the functions of the car well and is an expert driver, then the car will perform splendidly. If, on the other hand, a clumsy driver gets in the driver's seat, then no matter how impressive the vehicle's performance specs are, good driving will not be the outcome.

In addition, even though performance will vary by the auto model, if a skillful driver gets behind the wheel of even a car with inferior performance, he might well end up doing better than a poor driver does, who is driving a high performance car. In addition, how a car is utilized and whether or not it is well maintained will determine whether it will run smoothly or will need to be put in the shop.

The same holds true for bodily illnesses. For example,

even if you have a car that might easily break down, if you bring it in for the proper service checks, then you will end up without many mechanical problems. Likewise, even if you have a body that is genetically predisposed to illness, if you are careful enough, you might not become sick.

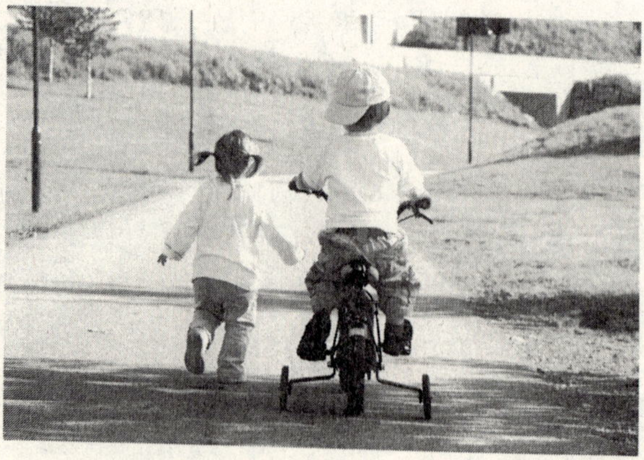

3
Invest for Health, Save Up Your Strength

Even though some religious people might be surprised, I would say that in order to guarantee a healthy lifestyle, the first thing you must do is to set aside some money. This is vital. It is important to spend an adequate amount of money on your health. If you try to cut corners on this point, it will cost you more in the long run.

You should consider an investment in your health as a mandatory expense. Think of it as fuel that your locomotive absolutely needs in order to run. In other words, as the basis of your thinking, you should hold to the concept that spending money for the sake of health is a good act. Out of your monthly income, how much are you currently putting towards maintaining your health?

White-collar workers in our cities get up early and get home late after a night of drinking, and are more than well aware that they do not get enough exercise. In fact, many seem to be plumping up like broiler chickens.

Such a person is not likely to regret the money he spends on gambling, drinking and other forms of socializing. However, how much money does he spend on exercise? Maybe that is something he should ask himself.

Oddly, people don't realize this way of looking at things. In fact, although people might give some consideration to how much exercise they have done, they do not give much thought to how much money they have spent for the sake of their personal health. Accordingly, it is possible to manage one's health by thinking this way. For example, say, you have a monthly income of 3,000 dollars; it may be appropriate to spend up to ten percent or 300 dollars of it for the sake of a healthy lifestyle. Let us draw up a budget to get a breakdown on exactly what these 300 dollars should be used for.

You could spend those 300 dollars each month in several ways. You can go to a gym and work out or swim. The white-collar worker's favored pastime of golf is another option. Cheaper activities include walking and jogging. However, even if forms of exercise that cost nothing are the best for your health, they are usually not pleasurable and people cannot continue long. That is the sticking point. This also holds true for other activities such as jumping rope. Therefore, people with the financial means must first resolve to devote a certain portion of their monthly income on their health.

Of course, if the individual concerned has a job that primarily involves manual labor and therefore is in good shape, it is probably OK for him to spend his money on something else. Here he might look to spend his money for relaxing the body rather than moving the body. Another option might be spending that money on some delicacy that he normally would not eat. In any case, as a first step, please resolve to set aside a definite portion of your income for the sake of a healthy lifestyle.

Of course, there are people who cannot spend much money. These people should resolve to spend time on their health instead.

For example, they might decide to get up thirty minutes early and exercise, or to devote a few hours on Saturday or Sunday to staying fit. There are many forms of exercise, which do not cost anything. In principle, you should begin with walking. There are other options, which require some form of equipment, such as jumping rope, swinging around a baseball bat or practicing your golf swing.

If you are going to stick with a form of exercise that is free, it is important that you get together with one or more exercising friends. The reason why you want to work out with friends is that it is just so easy for an individual's willpower to flag. Here, a cooperative attitude is important.

4
It All Begins with Walking

If you have not been getting enough exercise, then I would recommend that you begin with walking.

Those living in the city often find it difficult to set aside a place and time for walking, and in many cases, it boils down to the time they are commuting to and from work. However, if they can walk enough, their mental functions will be energized. This is a basic form of exercise.

For example, every day I carry a pedometer. Before going to sleep, I always record in a notebook how many steps I took during that particular day. I also weigh myself three times a day—in the morning, in the evening and at night. In fact, I do not just weigh

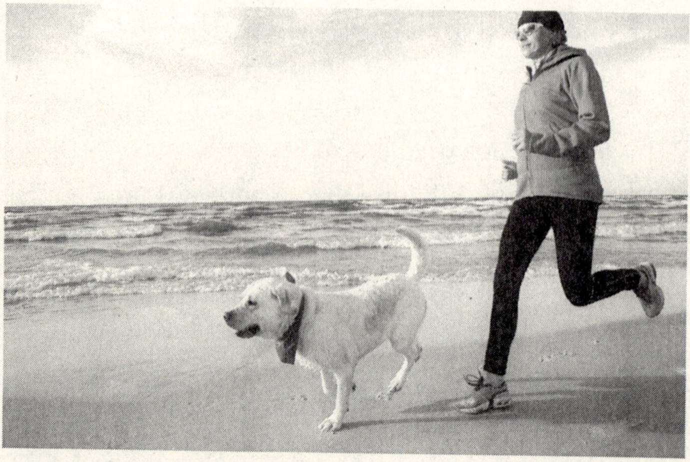

myself; I record my body fat ratio as well. Even at the same weight, if the amount of fat increases, this means that the amount of muscle has conversely declined. Therefore, if you maintain the same weight, but reduce your body's fat ratio, then the overall proportion of muscle will increase. I strive to control the tone of my body too.

In the past, I paid absolutely no attention to this. When I had many events that demanded the expenditure of strength, I would eat many energy-rich foods; since rest was the only way to recuperate from exhaustion, I would then rest up. However, if you rest after eating energy-packed foods, you are inviting weight gain. It is a matter of course. I have lost a lot of weight since I reached my peak weight, though; I managed to do so thanks to persistent effort and intentional control.

When I was still in my thirties and my body was still young and strong, I tended to think that I would never get sick. However, ever since I turned forty, I have become conscious of problems on the health front and now think about how to maintain good health.

I have also begun to think: "I don't want to cause a lot of trouble for people. In order to continue my work for a long time, I have to be proactive and do what needs to be done." As a result, I have been taking adequate steps to control my weight, not just to get thinner, but also to improve my physical strength.

Therefore, I started by walking 10,000 steps a day, and then tried exercises that demanded a bit more muscle power. I played tennis and swam, and rode my bicycle to train my legs. I also trained my muscles with dumbbells as well.

When you are in your teens or twenties, you do not realize much about the relationship between physical strength and the power to think. However, the fact is if you want to be able to continue studying for a long time, then you must maintain your physical strength.

5
A Surprising Method for Dissolving Worries

There is something special I would like to say in regards to the key to a healthy lifestyle. It has to do with a simple technique for warding off fatigue. The majority of people's worries are in fact due to fatigue.

If you have a healthy body that makes you bright-eyed and capable of enjoying a delicious breakfast when you get up in the morning, then even if you encounter problems during your day, in most cases it will not take much time to find solutions to them.

If, on the other hand, you are the kind of person who finds that it is difficult to get up in the morning, that breakfast does not taste good and that meeting people makes you feel out of sorts, then any problems that you happen to encounter will seem as giant obstacles. You will find yourself in a real fix. That is why finding ways to prevent fatigue is essential if you wish to remove your worries.

There are several methods for avoiding fatigue. A study of how the body operates shows that if it is provided with a certain amount of rest, it will be able to work more efficiently.

People usually cannot concentrate for more than an hour at a stretch. Even people with great concentration can only maintain it for two or three hours. After three hours, concentration quickly dissipates.

Nowadays, the number of people engaged in office work has grown enormously. However, if you do office work from morning until night, it is only natural that your efficiency will decline. I would make the conservative estimate that mental concentration can be sustained for only about an hour. I believe that in order to enjoy an hour of concentration, we need a small break of about five minutes. Therefore, the kind of thinking we must have is that for every hour we

Part 1 Chapter 1

How to Live a Healthy Lifestyle

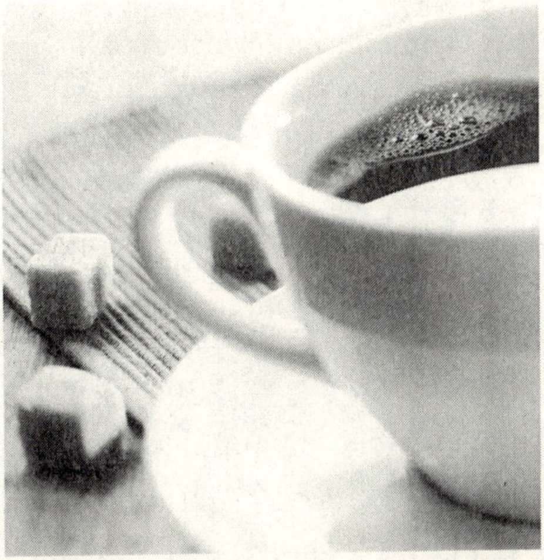

should put in fifty-five minutes of work that demands concentration and leave five minutes to relax the nerves.

Moreover, during your lunch break, if your office has a place where you can lie down or a sofa on which you can relax, then I think it is important that you should rest your body without any hesitation.

If you want to continue working all day for a long period, there are two parts of the body to which you should devote special care.

The first is the waist. If you feel pain in the area around your waist—including the hips and the small of the back—then your endurance will subsequently decline. Furthermore, you will lose your power of concentration. That is why you must practice stretching your torso. It is good to do light exercises during your lunch break to stretch out your waist; or, if you have the opportunity, you should stretch out on a sofa, or find some other way to unwind and relax.

The second area of importance is the feet. People weigh dozens of kilograms, but the soles of the feet cover only a very limited surface area. When such great weight is concentrated in such a small surface area, it is difficult to stand continuously for more than an hour. Actually, we tend to stand for several hours at a stretch in various positions. Therefore it is important to relax yourself. It is also important to set aside as much time as possible during which you can keep the weight off your feet. Remember, pay special attention to the waist and feet.

Another important consideration is how you use your eyes. If you read or perform similar activities over a long period, your eyes are certain to become tired. When your eyes are tired, it affects your brain and your stomach, making you nervous. As a result, you may develop a persecution complex regarding various things.

Therefore, you must find a way to minimize eyestrain as much as possible. In that regard, lighting is very important. It is also vital to keep a distance of twenty centimeters or more between written materials and your eyes. In addition, it would probably be wise to avoid small print as much as possible. If you have the choice of two formats for the same book, it would be

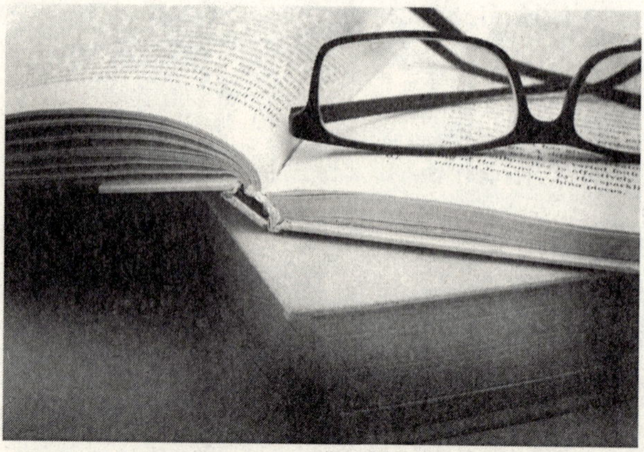

better to pay more for the hardcover edition rather than the pocketsize paperback with tiny print. In other words, you need to make a special effort so that your eyes will not worsen over the long term. Incidentally, we at Happy Science pay particular attention to layouts in order to help make our publications easy on the eyes.

Problems with the eyes are an obstacle that must be tackled for those that live an intellectual lifestyle. Please think of different ways to be able to continue making full use of your eyes.

The situation for the eyes is the same as those for the waist and feet. It is important that after you use them for a certain length of time you should look away for a bit to rest your eyes. Rather than using them continuously for five or ten hours, it is best to rest them a bit after one hour, and then if you use them again for an hour, take another short rest. If you do it this way, you should be able to keep using your eyes for more than eight to ten hours.

Waist, legs and eyes—pay careful attention to these three parts of the body in order to prevent fatigue.

The Mind and the Brain

Modern medicine says that once the brain is dead so is the human being. In short, once the functions of the brain come to a complete stop, then the person becomes a corpse. However, let us take a closer look at this.

I have been active as a religious leader for more than twenty years now. Moreover, it has also been more than two decades since my spiritual consciousness unfolded and I became capable of communicating with spirits in the other world who have already departed this Earth.

During this period, I have put out many volumes of spiritual messages. I have put in print what many famous historical figures have been thinking and philosophizing about since they entered the spirit world, and as books, these pronouncements have reached much of the world.

Judging from many of these actual experiences, I can state that people do not think with their brains. Even after they have been cremated in a crematorium, deceased people continue to adhere to the same habits and ways of thinking as when they were alive, and they are able to develop their own individual thoughts. They continue to have this capability after their deaths. This is the truth. I know this as the truth. People do not think with their brains. The brain is where computer-like functions or control functions are located. You might call it the "control room."

For that reason, people whose "machines," known as the brain, have become damaged are unable to make their thinking and conceptions known to the outside world, or to express themselves physically. Nevertheless, even though damage has been done to this function, it does not by any means signify that these people have completely lost their ability to think and conceptualize.

I believe that this is the most fundamental counterargument to the idea of brain death. In other words, human beings have a nerve center for thought in their souls, and their spiritual bodies. These continue to exist regardless of whether the

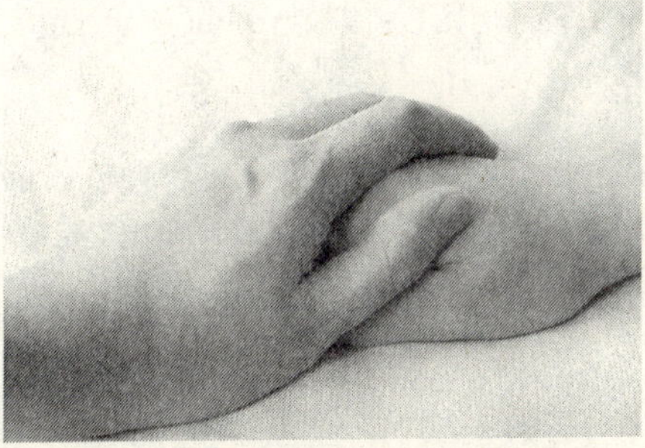

physical body lives or dies. This soul is the true form of the human being, and the physical body is nothing more than a "vehicle" for it.

It is just as if the physical body is the car and the soul is the driver. Just because the car is damaged does not mean that the driver has died. If a car breaks down and stops functioning, it will look as though the driver has stopped functioning as well. Yet, the life of the driver is a separate issue from the car. The car may be broken, but the driver is alive and well inside. We can say that the relationship between the soul and physical body is very similar to this analogy.

Furthermore, it would not be correct to say that people do not have the power to think and they cannot hear anything just because their brain is not responding. A spiritual body can read the minds of people around him without the function of the physical ear.

Consequently, people with terminal illnesses are capable of understanding what the people around them are saying and thinking.

Part I Chapter 2

The Spiritual Truth about Mind and Body

1 Meditation Prevents Cancer

Although improper diet and a lack of exercise can play important roles in causing disease, it can also be said that all modern illnesses arise from stress. Especially in the case of internal organs, most of the illnesses are caused by stress. Doctors attribute various causes to illnesses, but if you investigate further, it all narrows down to stress.

People today do not live a harmonious, truth-oriented lifestyle. Because in most cases they move in business circles or some other worldly society with bad vibrations, they are always forced to endure some kind of worry. For example, if a person makes a major blunder at work and he is strongly admonished by his boss or if a payment slip is not honored and the company finds itself in a bind, he is likely to become a nervous wreck. What happens then?

Not only does every physical body contain an identically shaped spiritual body, every organ has its own corresponding spiritual body part. So a physical heart has a spiritual heart, a physical liver has a spiritual liver and a physical stomach has a spiritual stomach and so forth.

Each of these spiritual body parts has a different way of feeling things because they have their own special mission and unique ways of working. For example, the spiritual body of the stomach is extremely sensitive, and its sense of feeling is very acute. The heart feels various things on a larger scale.

In this manner, the spiritual bodies of the various organs are symbolic of various things. Therefore, if human beings generate great amounts of stress, in accordance with the nature of the stress involved, the spiritual bodies of the internal organs are the first to suffer damage.

Also since the physical functions including internal organs are closely related to the spiritual bodies, when the spiritual body is damaged, the illness will start to appear on the physical body as well.

The same holds true when a person is diagnosed with cancer. First, some kind of problem arises with the spiritual body of an organ, and after that an abnormality appears in the physical body. This is a form of possession. Although it is only a partial possession, the root cause can be traced back to stress. Therefore, please be aware that it is of the utmost importance to live with a harmonious mind in the midst of third-dimensional waves.

Although there are cases in which a body becomes out of shape because of physical causes, more often than not, the greater probability is that stress causes worse damage. It is better to prevent this stress in order for most people to live a healthy lifestyle.

The principle of love and the principle of self-reflection are what we need to prevent this stress. In addition, meditation and positive thinking help. Happy

Science has methods of meditating. When we meditate, we relax our various internal organs as well as our nerve system, which helps in preventing diseases that come from stress.

In particular, it is the best method for preventing cancer. Since in nearly all cases cancer can be attributed to stress, I would recommend meditation as a preventive measure.

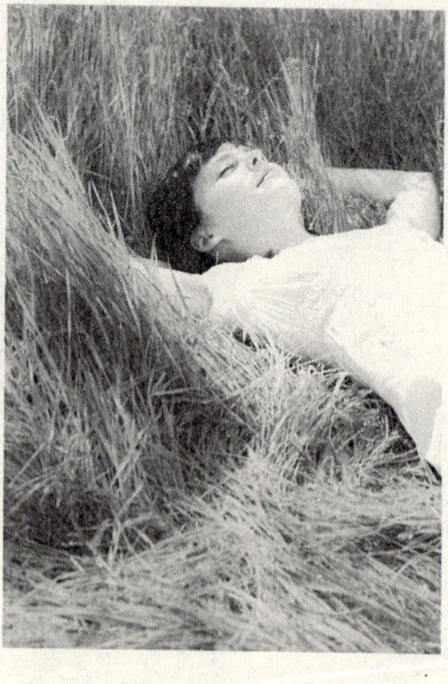

2

Let Go of Hatred and Learn to Forgive

In most cases people, who become ill with an unknown cause, often have strong feelings of hatred. If you hate other people, then your physical condition will degenerate. People who are hated are likely to be in poor condition, but so too are those who hate. If you do not forgive and continue to harbor feelings of dislike, the workings of your mind develop nests of diseases within your body. Destructive thoughts and ill will materialize into cancer cells.

In this manner, even without being aware of it, you find that a disease has developed within your body. Consequently, if you have been thinking something like, "I will hate that person as long as I am alive," it is important to step back and think: "If I continue to hate him, then I am certain to suffer too. So I should forgive him."

You must forgive others for your own sake. Not only must you forgive yourself for things you have done, you must also forgive others for things they have done. Without a doubt, there are people who have harmed you, who have brought shame upon you, who have persecuted you, and who have humiliated you. Surely, there are many such individuals. Yet you must forgive them. If the suffering has already lasted for a year, or three or five years, then surely the time has come to let it go.

Such people may have changed already, and may be engaging in self-reflection too. There could be cases where the person may have treated you with contempt, but reflected on their deed later on. So, there is no reason for continuing to hate them. Even if someone has done something awful to you, which has left bitter memories, you must not hold onto vengeful thoughts forever, but should instead think, "Well, that person is imperfect, just like me."

3
Past Lives and Illnesses

There are many cases in which the ways a person died in past lives will have considerable effect on the symptoms of illnesses that appear in this life.

If the soul is stamped with experiences of deep injury and suffering because of illnesses or accidents that caused death in past lives, then the suffering will begin to show even though the person has a new body this time around. In many cases, the exterior portion of the spiritual body—the astral body—will undergo changes, which will eventually manifest themselves in the physical body.

Influences from Past Lives

Example 1. People with Distinctive Birthmarks

For example, when a person has a distinctive birthmark on his body, in many instances it closely corresponds to the way in which that person died in a past life.

Many cases have been reported of marks being located on the same parts of the body where in past lives people were killed by swords or spears, or died after being hit by arrows. In effect, they are reminders that the person died in such a way in the past.

Example 2. People with Skin Diseases, Asthma or Bronchitis

With skin diseases, there are of course cases in which allergies develop as a result of personal relations. As taught in Happy Science, if we trace back into the past lives of people with skin problems we find that there are also many cases in which they are connected to the way the person died in a past life.

In the case of a person who was burned to death,

since the skin will strongly retain the sensation of being burned by fire, when that person is born into this life, corresponding birthmarks will sometimes appear. There are many other cases in which the connection manifests itself in various forms of skin disease or terrible skin allergies.

Even if they died in the same situation from a fire, there are also people who painfully suffocated to death because of the smoke. These people may suffer from asthma, bronchitis or some other form of disease of the respiratory system in this life.

Through regressive hypnosis, people can find out how they had died in a past life and how it has manifested in this life time. In many cases, these illnesses will be healed when the individuals realize this connection. This is a truly "scary" fact.

Since the symptoms appear on the body because there is a cause in the mind, if the mind is corrected, then the outside too will be healed. In this way, it is true that people with lingering memories of their deaths in a past life, who suffered terribly and were enveloped by smoke, may have asthma in the present life.

Example 3. People Who Fear Water

Then again there are people who are terrified of water. These people think, "I'm scared of going into the water. Swimming pools scare me to death. I'm also scared of rivers. Anyhow, I can't avoid being horrified when I see water."

In most cases, a spiritual reading reveals that such a person experienced a water-related death in a past life. This experience of death by water may have taken any number of forms, including drowning, an accident in the water, being murdered in water, or dying in a flood.

In such cases, their souls will likely be engraved with incredible terror. Such a feeling of terror in the soul might appear in a form of phobia in this life too. Therefore it is no wonder that they should have a fear of water.

Example 4. People Who Fear Heights

An even more common example is acrophobia, or fear of heights. When people suffering from this phobia go up to a high place, they will be absolutely unable to control their fears. But if we conduct spiritual readings of such people's past lives, in nearly every case, we find that they died after falling from a high place.

That may happen in war, or by falling, or by being pushed off cliffs, shoved from roofs, from turrets, from windows of buildings, or otherwise from suffering an experience of falling during a past life. In such cases, these people cannot help their fear of high places.

Recently, there are cases where people who died in airplane accidents were reborn, and now have a fear of airplanes. These people are scared to death of boarding an airplane.

In this manner, a soul will carry over various things from past lives, and experiences of fear in past lives will resurface.

If someone experiences a major accident in this life, it remains as karma and so the next time that person is reborn, it is likely that a fear of it will develop (see p.72, "The Truth about Mind and Body 2").

Example 5. People Who Fear Enclosed Spaces

There are also people who suffer from claustrophobia or fear of enclosed spaces. Take the case of a person who says: "I'm terrified of enclosed places. Small rooms are scary to me, and elevators are intimidating too. I'm terrified if the doors are locked. In other words, I feel like I'm suffocating." Spiritual readings of past lives will likely show that these people died in such a manner. Such people were killed under circumstances in which they were trapped and could not escape.

For example, if a person died in a Nazi gas chamber, in this life such an individual will be absolutely terrified of being trapped in an enclosed area. In cases like it, in which large numbers of people died, the deceased are reborn relatively quickly, but a very great percentage of them will retain this fear.

If we do a spiritual reading much farther back into the past, we can find cases in which the cause of such a fear of enclosed places can be traced all the way back to ancient Egypt.

In ancient Egypt, when a pharaoh died, his servants

and handmaidens were buried alive along with the pharaoh's jewels and treasures inside the pyramid or other graves. The reason why they were buried alive was because people thought, "When the pharaoh arrives in the next world, he will be inconvenienced if he finds himself all alone. Since the pharaoh will surely face difficulties in his everyday life, let's send his servants along with him into the next world." Thus, these servants were buried alive and allowed to die.

In such cases, no doubt these people were not yet ready to die. As a result it became karma and gave rise to their fear of enclosed spaces or the terror of being buried alive.

Example 6. People Who Suffer from Panic Disorder

There are also cases in which, in a past life, when a person was walking in the mountains, out of the blue he was set upon and killed by brigands, or was slain in a surprise attack, or was cut down by thieves in a back alley, or had his home invaded by robbers who had finished him off, or was otherwise murdered without warning. When a person who experienced this is reborn, a variety of extremely anxious feelings and terrors will be present, and he is likely to develop a panic disorder.

In this way, if you cannot find enough evidence of the cause in this life, even if you look back to your youth, it is quite likely that abnormal experiences in one of your many past lives are at work.

For hints on how to overcome such suffering, please also refer to the answers in "Overcoming Past Trauma" in Part II, Chapter 1, "Healing Your Mind."

4

You Have the Power to Regenerate

Human beings have the ability to restore their own bodies. However, they have forgotten this fact to a large extent, and thus this ability remains dormant.

For example, looking at the natural world, lizards are able to regenerate their tails if they lose their original ones. There are crabs that can re-grow their pincers if they are torn off. Crabs use their pincers for defense and also to get food, so if they lose them, they will not be able to survive. These scissor-like appendages have a rather complex structure and this power to regenerate them is bestowed by God.

This is to say nothing of the fact that human beings, who are so much more beloved by God, certainly have

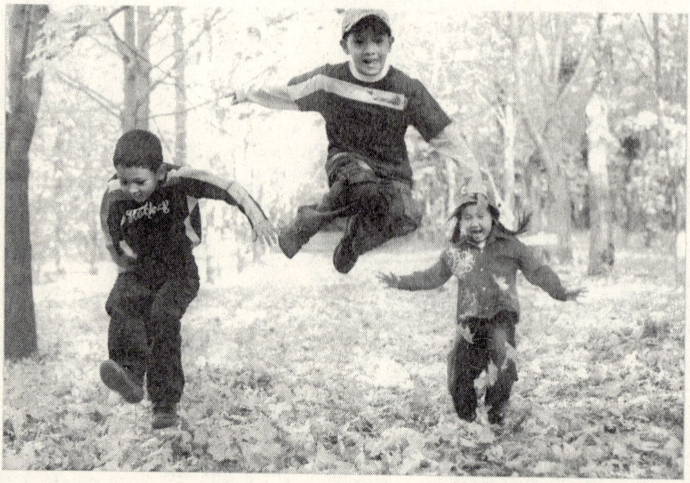

the innate ability to restore a part of the body, if they truly wish to become healthy. The reason why they cannot is because human beings have become quite poisoned by materialism, and they think that such things are impossible.

Doctors usually say, "A person can move his voluntary muscles with his willpower, but since the internal organs are involuntary muscles it cannot be moved with his willpower." Since that is what the textbooks say, it is probably engraved in your brains. But that is not the way things actually are.

The human body is made up of bones, like the skull, and internal muscles, which all change to some degree through life. It may take time, but there is nothing that does not undergo change. Consequently, if you strongly maintain the wish to heal your body, then even if the process is slow, many things can in fact be healed.

Since the strength of your thoughts can change your body for the worse and even cause cancers to form, surely you also have the capability of using it in a positive direction.

There are people who have weak stomachs, hearts, livers or other internal organs, but the functioning of such internal organs can also change. They can become stronger. In cases where the brain is weak, the problem is a little more difficult. Still, the brain can also be made stronger even though studying and other strategies are necessary.

It is best to believe that the bodies of human beings can be cured in this manner. Although it may take some time, if you strongly believe in this fashion, then the healing can indeed take place.

During that interval, it is necessary that you undertake measures for the sake of your own health. If you do nothing except pray for healing, it will likely be in vain. You must be very conscientious about doing your part. For example, if you are smoking one hundred cigarettes a day and pray, "Please cure me of lung cancer," it would certainly be a selfish attitude. You really need to live up to your end of the bargain.

If you have high cholesterol, there is no alternative but to bring it down. You must cut down on your intake of high cholesterol foods, get more exercise, and put forth all necessary effort while you also maintain strong healing thoughts. This is how change will appear. Since all kinds of things like this can happen, strive to make the power of your thinking a bit stronger.

Nowadays, many young people are wearing braces on their teeth, as many of them desire to have their teeth straightened. But actually teeth can move by themselves. Spend about a year thinking strongly of their moving, and they will start to move. If you think, "This one will have to move about five millimeters," and continue to think like that, the tooth will move.

The same holds true for your eyes. God did not endow human beings with useless bodies with eyes that are destined to become near-sighted. However, once you start wearing glasses, the eyes get accustomed to it, and the eye muscles no longer move the way you want them to. That is all there is to it. You are originally able to move the lenses of your eyes.

The various parts of the human body are given room for growth and development. Consequently, they have the ability to heal illnesses. Although this process may take a bit of time, I am confident that a combination of thoughts and actions can result in healing.

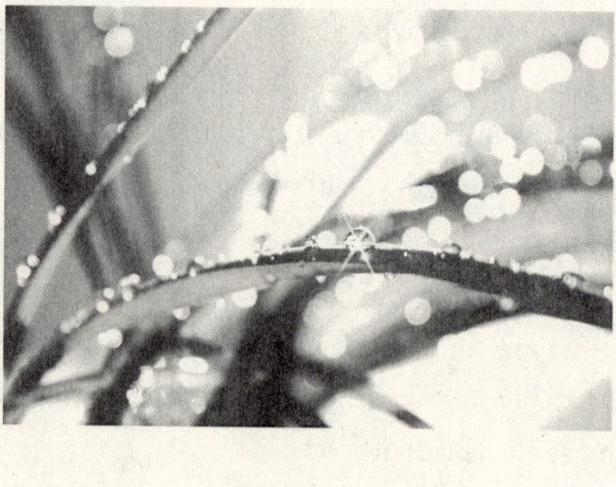

5
The Truth of Organ Transplants

Organs are not merely material in nature. They are also accompanied by consciousnesses. In fact, organs have spiritual consciousnesses too.

The heart is the spiritual center where the intentions and feelings of human beings are concentrated. If the heart is removed from someone's body without their complete understanding and consent, and is subsequently transplanted into another person's body, then part of the heart's spiritual body will be transplanted as well.

In this manner, when a heart is transplanted to another body, and when the donor has not yet accepted his own death, spiritual possession takes place. The donor's soul is pulled by his own heart and moves into the new body, giving rise to spiritual possession. That is to say, the soul of the person who is receiving the transplant, and the soul that has taken possession of him, enters into a state of co-existence within the body. As a result, we might see rejection reactions or other complications. There are many examples reported in the past in which a powerful rejection follows the transplant of an organ.

Moreover, when this happens, and souls are prevented from making the journey to the other world, these souls will, in many cases, become stray spirits because of their dissatisfaction or attachment to this world.

These spirits have the power to make all kinds of interference and bad developments to take place, so that one unlucky event after the next might occur within the family of the person that received the organ transplant. This problem has, since ancient times, been referred to as a "haunting." This is the truth from the spiritual perspective.

When I see heart surgeons conducting heart transplants, it brings something specific to mind: the ancient civilization of the Maya.

In the ancient Mayan empire there was a rite in which hearts were torn out of living human beings and offered to the gods. I have heard that tens of thousands or even hundreds of thousands of people had their hearts torn out of them, while they were still alive, for use as sacrificial offerings to the gods.

It seems to me that many of today's heart surgeons had professions like these priests in the age of the ancient Mayan civilization, who wielded knives, and tore out the hearts of millions. Perhaps they are reincarnations of the very same people.

In addition, it seems to me that the heart transplants are more akin to ancient religious rituals than cutting-edge science. Isn't medicine still at an unenlightened stage? I believe that as long as we do not recognize the connection between the body and the soul, we will find it impossible to move past the stage of amateurish medical treatment. The spiritual bodies of human beings can feel sensations of pain. But most physicians do not seem to realize that when terminally ill patients receiving intravenous drip treatments die, their spiritual bodies still suffer from the pain of the needles stuck in their arms.

Even more so, it is hard to imagine the degree of suffering that a spiritual body is subjected to if organs are removed while a person is in a "brain dead" state. You should all be aware that modern medicine is still languishing in an uncivilized stage.

6
Why Is Your Physical Body Mortal?

The world beyond ours is in fact the real world, while this world is only temporary. This world exists as a place for people to undergo training for their souls. In this sense, this world is not totally imaginary. This world is a place where the soul borrows the temporary form of flesh for the sake of self-expression.

Be that as it may, a physical body must inevitably enter the path of decline. Therefore, even if you pursue happiness in this world, that will not be a final form of happiness. It is important to pursue happiness that will continue from this world to the next. This is the happiness that comes from "enlightenment."

For example, if we say that Shakyamuni Buddha did

not seek happiness for himself, that would not be true. In a Buddhist sutra, Shakyamuni Buddha declares, “There is no man who has sought happiness more than I.” In fact, Shakyamuni Buddha continuously searched for the happiness of enlightenment.

In short, as long as people are attached to the bodily portion, or the temporary portion of this world, ultimate happiness cannot be achieved. This world is a world of flux in which all things are transient, and nothing is permanent. Human beings cannot remain young and beautiful forever. As we grow older, our hair turns white, we get hunched over at the waist, and our faces become wrinkled. Eventually we become ill and die. Birth, Aging, Illness and Death were unavoidable 2,500 years ago and still is today.

Modern medicine is constantly striving to lengthen our life spans, yet they remain finite. Rather, we are now subject to sufferings that were not around 2,500 years ago. Measures taken in terminal medical treatment require many tubes to be stuck into patients' bodies—this is called the “spaghetti syndrome,” and I believe a life passed under such conditions can only be one of suffering.

In that sense, we can say that new forms of suffering have arisen for the sake of lengthening life spans. That is because medicine itself does not recognize the world after death, and it considers life in this world to be all that we have.

As far as life in this world is concerned, it is important to live, as happily as possible, but after passing a certain point, we should be willing to wind things up. After all, this world is nothing more than a

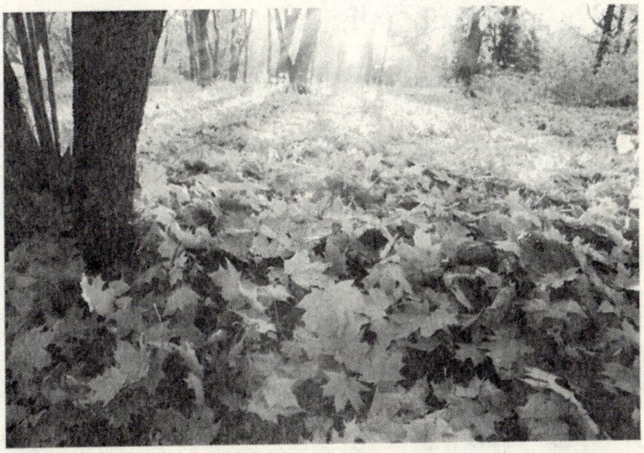

stop on the way to the next world.

For example, even if elementary school was a supremely happy world for us, we cannot remain a primary school student forever. Although at the time we might have cried while saying, "I don't want to say goodbye to my friends," we will have to part with dear friends as we move on up to middle school, and then eventually high school, and to college.

Although partings can be bitter, if we do not experience them, we are not able to develop to the next step. Human beings living on this earth must all pass through the gateway of death and experience separations from family and friends. Then, in accordance with our achievements in this world, we will go to the next world, a place where our comrades will be. It is similar to the way in which we progress through junior high school, high school and finally college, based on our individual academic abilities.

Accordingly, it will not do good to regret separations. To the end, it is best to have ingrained the feeling that all things are transient.

7
Lessons from the Severely Disabled and Ill

Today's Japan is excessively wealthy, resulting in "diseases of affluence," contempt for others, and vaulting ambitions; most people, though, are not even aware that they have become infected with an illness of the mind. I would like such people to return to the starting point of humankind and to give consideration to what their model should be.

There are also many people in this world who have not been blessed. There are poor people and sick people, as well as individuals who were born with disabilities. You may feel sorry for their plight, but at the same time such people serve as teachers whose message is, "What happiness it must be to have been born with a sound body or into a well-off family."

It is not that their soul itself is evil nor is it that they were born like that to be punished under the Law of Karma, as it used to be interpreted in ancient India.

In the midst of our affluent society, such unfortunate people are teaching others that they should not act mistakenly, or stray from the right path; these people also point out the mistakes of the mind that have been made. By showing us the problems that exist, the disabled and the unfortunate in fact provide guidance for others.

The ranks of unfortunates are swollen with children

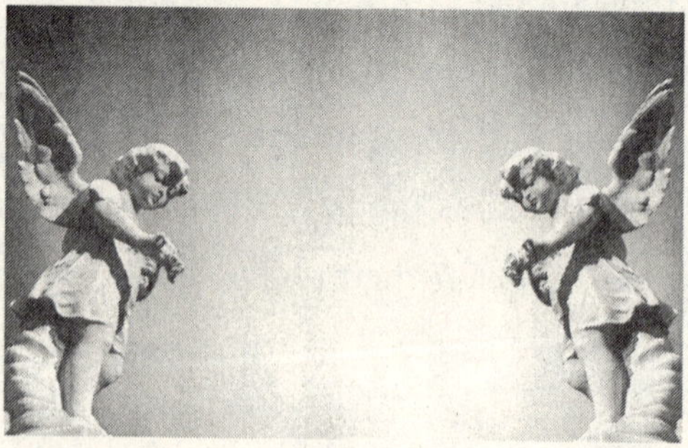

with severe disabilities, people with incurable diseases, and individuals who must rely on people's care in their daily lives. These people could be Bodhisattvas of compassion in disguise. There are many people with this mission. Among them are individuals like Helen Keller, who lived a life that had an enormous influence on the world.

And on a smaller scale, there are other people who live in poverty or suffering, so that their existence might admonish arrogant people and afford them an opportunity to awaken.

In present-day Japan, many people do not take notice of the fact that such people are really their teachers. And being ignorant of the fact that these special ones were born to act as teachers, many people look down on them, treat them as fools, make fun of them, or feel nothing whatsoever concerning them. I believe that this is a cause for shame.

How about devoting a bit more concrete attention to really considering what love is? And then do what you can to put it into practice.

The Truth about Mind and Body 2

Life Is Like a Workbook

It is often said that, "All men are created equal," but if you look at different people, it is easy to feel that there are actually extreme gaps in their respective states in life. They differ both on the outside and inside.

Where is the starting point for these differences? It is not to be found in this life alone. Human beings go through reincarnations eternally, and the accumulation of previous lives is influencing this life. Each human being has karma, a concept that has come to be comparatively well-known today.

Although karma rightfully has both a good side and bad side, in most cases the concept is viewed mainly in a negative sense. For example, this thinking is expressed in the following statements: "You are being hurt by others in this life, because in your past life you hurt other people," "You have lost your sight in this life because in a past life you put out someone else's eyes," or "You have a bad leg in this life because you injured someone's leg in a past life."

There is a tendency to think that the karmic law of cause and effect accumulates and manifests in this life. If we do a life reading of someone, and examine that person's past lives, the fact is that with a certain degree of probability, we can say that there is such a correlation. So if we think of life as a workbook, the most significant problem contained therein concern not just what has arisen in this life but in many cases also the causal actions in past lives.

However, this concept of karma should not be approached solely from the standpoint of "merits rewarded and sins punished." True enough, someone who committed homicide in a past life may well find a murderous end to his current life. Nevertheless, that is not necessarily a punishment. When a person is reborn, he chooses the life he will live. Since some people become enlightened only through experience, such souls in fact choose a harsh environment in which to be born.

In this manner, we can see that the plan of life does not contain only good things. It also includes the necessary processes for your soul to grow and develop to the highest degree. People who plan such lives are well aware of the difficulties they will face.

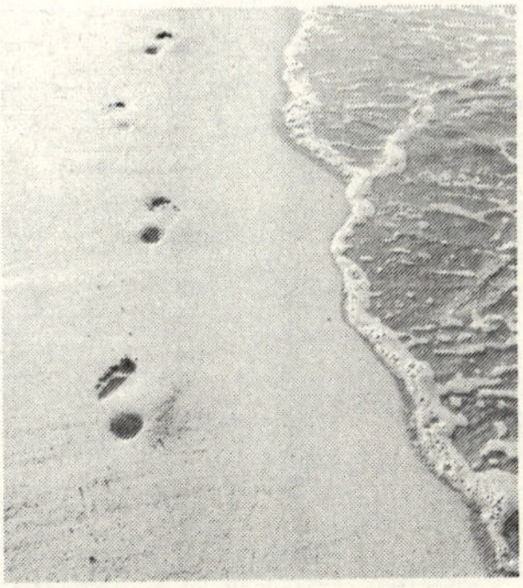

Part II

Q&A Effective Advice for Mind and Body

Part II Chapter 1

Healing Your Mind

1

Remedies for Mild Depression

Q: Many people are suffering from mild depression these days. Please explain what the causes of and countermeasures for mild depression are as seen from a spiritual perspective.

A: First, if we consider what the causes of this condition are, we find that in many cases it is because some spiritual influence is at work.

However, what I would like you to remember here is that the being that is possessing or influencing a person, and the person being influenced are both on the same spiritual wavelength.

In such situations, various kinds of spirits are

attracted but if we look at the kinds of spirits that appear, we can tell in an instant which part of the person's mind is ill. An entity with no spiritual connection will not appear. Always and without fail, there will be some kind of familiarity. This is a fundamental principle.

Consequently, if the person finds himself subjected to some kind of spiritual interference, he must look back at himself to make sure that within his mind there is nothing that invites these spirits.

Remedy for Mild Depression 1 — Calmly Reflect on Your Mind

When you are in this situation, the teaching of self-reflection will have the greatest effect. Self-reflection is the royal road to recovery. So, quietly reflect back on your mind.

When outside spirits are nearby or when a person is prone to spiritual interferences, the most common response would be the tendency to blame things on somebody else. Right off the bat, you put the blame on others. Inevitably, you start to say, "That person did wrong," or, "It's his fault."

If this tendency manifests itself, consider carefully whether it is indeed your own opinion. Is it your own idea, or did the idea emanate from someone else who has gotten you to think that way? You need to consider this point calmly.

Before blaming things on someone else, first calm your mind, and then check to ensure that you do not have any problems lurking within your own mind. Furthermore, if you do have any problems, it means you need to practice self-reflection; even if the process is time-consuming, you must go on removing each cloud from your mind. If you can repent well, then you will surely become stronger. Engaging in self-reflection is the first option.

Remedy for Mild Depression 2 — Don't Struggle, Wait for Time to Pass

Another method for dealing with mild depression when everything seems out of kilter is to refrain from struggling too much. At such a time, you are liable to think, "I have to do something right away." However, if you struggle too much, you will find yourself increasingly entangled in the trap.

A basic principle is that possession by evil spirits does not last for long. The reason for this is that the true place they belong is Hell. Hell is a world of tangled resentments, a world of delusions of persecution where everyone embraces ill will. Even if the inhabitants of that world temporarily possess people on earth, if they possess a person for a long period, they will also begin to suffer because the vibrations of Hell and of our world differ.

Although the person who is possessed suffers, so too, does the spirit that possesses. Please be aware of this fact. In particular, should the person who has been possessed engage in "the exploration of the right mind," then the possessing spirit will suffer considerably. Think of it this way: "I am suffering, but so too is the other side." Such a situation cannot last for very long.

Consequently, even a person who is not yet sufficiently awakened spiritually can usually expect to

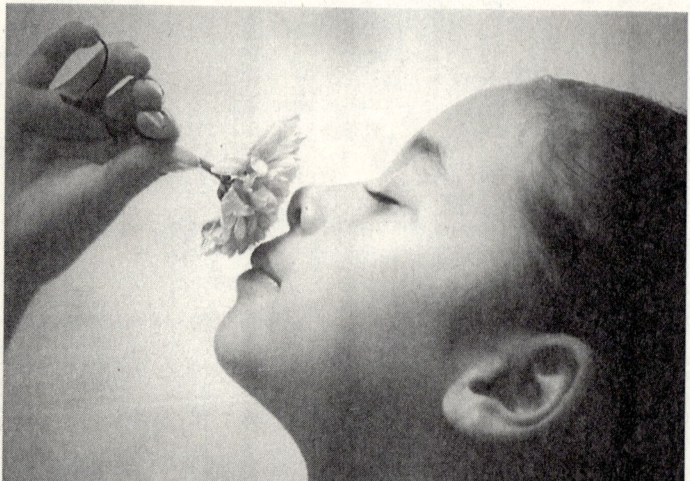

be released from the possession in about three months, or six months at the most. If a normal lifestyle is adopted, the possessing spirit will surely go away. In cases where possession has temporarily caused a mild depression, it does not last longer than this.

The reason why it does not continue is that the spirit's comrades in Hell are certain to come to take him back. They will try to pull him back saying, "How long are you thinking of having fun." That is why it will not last long.

So, please wait for time to pass. If, during that interval, you struggle and do something foolish, you will end up with undesirable results. So a little waiting is best. If you have the fortitude to wait half a year, I guarantee things will change for the better.

Remedy for Mild Depression 3
— Brace Yourself for the Worst

Another method is to switch over to positive thinking. If you are always thinking only about bad things, unavoidably you will become a prisoner of them. When you have a mild depression and are under strong spiritual influence, you tend to think of small negative things as if they were huge. An evil thing as small as a fingertip becomes monstrously large. In the mind of this individual, even small misfortunes often become a matter of life and death—towering problems with earth-shattering repercussions.

At such a time, it is necessary to revert to the state of a calm mind. If your mind calms down, then you should think, "Even if I lose my life, no one can take away my immortal soul."

Since the souls of people are immortal, there is actually nothing that can be taken away. We have immortal souls and eternal life. Life, in this sense, is not something that we can be deprived of. The worst possible thing that can happen is that you will lose your life in this world. Usually it is only a matter of your family relationships becoming difficult, being detested by other people, or being fired from your company.

However, no one can go so far as to take away your eternal life. Since that is impossible, you should try to imagine the worst possible outcome and brace yourself for the worst, thinking, "Even under these circumstances, I think I can continue living." If you brace yourself for the worst and make yourself ready, you will not be bewildered. Then, after strengthening your will in this way, if you wait for a bit, you will soon be able to see various "seeds of light."

Although up until that point you probably thought only of negative things, sure enough good things will begin to happen. There is no reason why negative things should continue unbroken. If you are willing to wait half a year, as one month or even two weeks pass by, good things will begin to happen, so try not to waste those opportunities.

You have to nurture these seeds. Pay close attention to the good things you did, the good things that happened and other happy events, and nurture these seeds so that they grow. Then, by expanding your happiness, your unhappiness will vanish. This method of lighting a candle to dispel the darkness is indeed a fine strategy.

Especially for people afflicted with mild depression, if it is difficult to battle with the negative parts of oneself, it would be better to use positive thinking. They should switch their ways of thinking by "looking only for the good."

We have been discussing what is generally recommended for people under spiritual influences to do. Then, what should you do if someone you know is in such a condition?

First, praise the good aspects of that person. Starting from this will guarantee maximum effects. If you criticize that person's bad points, he will only become that much more out of control. For that reason, make sure to begin with praise and cheerful talk.

It is important to embrace them with a harmonious atmosphere. This circle of friendship or supporting thoughts from friends is important. Even if a person cannot win out against evil spirits alone, if people gather round to help, then the evil spirits cannot win.

A person who looks solely on the dark side can find any amount of dark things. Nevertheless, people who look on the side of happiness, will find happy elements increasing. Please make efforts in this regard.

2
Harmful Influences of Dieting

Q: Many young women today are taking dieting too far, and I am concerned that this might exert a bad influence on their minds and bodies.

A: Dieting which is carried out in line with normal healthy methods is heavenly, and there is no special reason for worry. However, if a diet is unreasonable and food and drink are eliminated to an extreme degree, a person may end up being possessed by wandering souls from Hell that are known as "hungry spirits."

Nowadays, young women like to equate slimness with beauty, and many of them do indeed become as thin as rails. In order that they might be able to wear slender garments, they go without eating, surviving on little more than salads and juices, rapidly becoming thinner and thinner.

Nevertheless, even though they duly become thin, they often rebound to their former weight. After wasting away to a skeleton, they then go to the opposite extreme and eat constantly, so that although they might have lost ten kilograms, they end up twenty kilograms heavier than their initial weight. In this manner, if a person swings back and forth from weight loss to weight gain, it is best to conclude that a spirit influence is at work. In other words, she is possessed.

While there are human spirits in Hell, there are also many animal spirits, as well. The hells to which animals go are most often shallow worlds, and in nearly all cases they fall into Hell because they have starved to death, or because they were attacked and killed. Animals, which died due to an accident, starvation, from being eaten, from being killed, or the like cannot go to the heavenly realm, and thus end up in the Hell of Animals.

Some animal spirits come out of this Hellish world and approach human beings of this world. They tend to possess human beings, especially children, who are inordinately attached to food. When such a spirit possesses a person, it gives rise to an abnormal appetite.

If you are such a person as this, then it is important to thoroughly study Happy Science teachings, and to cultivate a cheerful spirit and self-control; in other words, your mind must be the master of yourself. You also have to discipline and make efforts to correct your lifestyle habits, thus engaging in a diligent lifestyle. Furthermore, as far as food is concerned, it is best to make efforts to control your eating within logical limits.

If you practice dieting within appropriate limits, then it will have no connection with Hell. If you go to extremes, though, the wandering spirits of Hell or animal spirits may well possess you.

Conversely, because of becoming possessed, you may find that you have developed an abnormal appetite or have become active at nighttime. Especially in cases where a person engages in round after round of gorging on food in the middle of the night followed by vomiting, it is best to conclude that in almost all instances this results from possession by an animal spirit which has fallen to the Hell of Hungry Spirits, or by a human spirit who has starved to death.

When you check yourself or have members of your family or someone else do the monitoring and find that your lifestyle is a bit abnormal, it is important to correct it. Abstinence, diligence, and discipline—if you wholeheartedly embrace these virtues I am confident that you will be able to escape any animalistic influences.

3
Sleeping Peacefully Without Spiritual Restraints

Q: Sometimes I have bad dreams that can be truly frightening nightmares or I experience the feeling that I am being tied down to my bed by restraints. What can I do to sleep soundly?

A: If you have terrible nightmares, we can conclude that in most cases an evil spirit is nearby. Likewise, if you feel shackled so that your sleeping body cannot move at all or it seems like a weight is pressing down on your chest, evil spirits have arrived to engage in various forms of mischief. If you are restrained like this in the middle of the night, let me offer some methods for escaping these situations.

Remedies for Spiritual Restraints
Step 1. **Prayer**

First, this can be solved by prayer, so the typical method for Happy Science members should be to look for help from me, our organization's supporting spirit group, and their guardian spirits through recitations of prayers such as: "Words of Truth: The Dharma of the Right Mind," "Prayer to the Lord," "Prayer for Exorcising Evil Spirits," and "Prayer to Guardian and Guiding Spirits" (Sutras limited for Happy Science members).

Additionally, the best thing to do if you are able to move your hand is to turn on the light and sleep with it on. Since it is easier for evil spirits to make their approach in a darkened room, you should try leaving your lamp on.

Also, try playing one of my lectures on CD or cassette tape, etc. If you do that, it will thoroughly displease the evil spirits and they will run away. If evil spirits have habitually possessed you, this should allow you to sleep well, and it works effectively for people who are attacked by evil spirits only at night. This is another method.

Step 2. Breathing Methods

Breathing methods offer another approach. If you cannot move and there is nothing you can do about it, in order to regain your own spirit, you should try catching your breath.

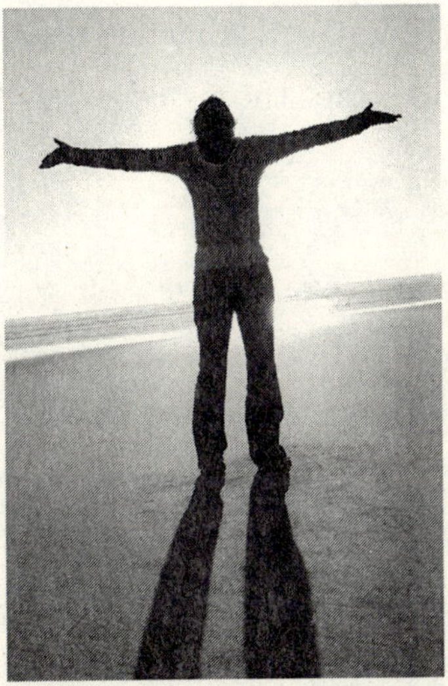

As you are lying down, try to breathe from the lower stomach area below the belly button. The idea is to provide your body with fresh oxygen. Try breathing in, and if you are able to repeat this deep respiration several times over, strangely enough you will find that the evil spirits have parted from you.

One of the secrets of this breathing method is that as you breathe, light will enter your body. When that happens, the evil spirits will float up and away from your body. Or else the hands of the evil spirits that are holding you down will let go. At that moment, you will be free.

This is how to escape through the breathing method.

Step 3. Positive Thinking and Self-Reflection

Another method is to change your perspective into a positive one. The fact that evil spirits can approach you is evidence that the wavelengths given off by your mind and the wavelengths of the evil spirits are the same, so in this case you should reverse the situation. You must eliminate any thinking about negative things and look towards the light. Think only about wonderful, positive things within your mind. This is another method for dealing with this threat.

Another strategy is to practice self-reflection. Even if the weight on your chest prevents your body from moving and you cannot move your hands either, that does not mean that this restraint is extending into your head. Therefore, while lying down, engage in self-reflection.

If you find yourself in such a situation, it means that at some point up to the prior day you have been having trouble with human relationships. In this situation, try thinking about the person with whom you get along the least, a person about whom you think, "I can't stand him", or, "If only she wasn't around." If there is someone in your life who fits this description, then try thinking of him or her and practice self-reflection. In any event, start with apologizing to this person.

Step 4. Giving Thanks

Next, another method is giving thanks.

One day is like a lifetime. If you live by this

philosophy, then the end of each day corresponds to the end of your entire life. So you should give thanks by saying something like this: "It is my turn to leave this world. Now I can return to a pleasurable world. Looking back over my life on this earth, I can say that I truly had a good life. Thank you so much. Even if I should die here and now, I am satisfied." By giving thanks like this, you will make the evil spirits feel stupid and that will drive them away. This is another method for dealing with the problem.

The next time you experience a bad dream, I suggest that you try out some of the methods explained above.

Only psychics can actually tell how it feels when evil spirits come and how it feels to get rid of them, but average people can also experience a similar situation if it is in their dreams. If evil spirits come—that is to say, if you have a bad dream, or experience the sensation of being pressed down and restrained, so that you recognize that they have "come"—then try each of the methods I have offered in the order in which I presented them. As you work through the methods, the job will be done.

4

Anxiety from Menstrual Period

Q: Women tend to feel emotionally unstable during their menstrual period. During such a time, how can a woman gain effective control of her own mind?

A: The reason why a woman has to shoulder the "handicap" of menstruation is because the experience offers something from which her soul can learn.

However, in approaching this problem, we need to go beyond thinking about menstruation in isolation, and instead must consider it as part of the chain process which links giving birth, raising, and feeding a child.

I believe it is because women have different handicaps

from men. No doubt about it, we can say that the fact that a woman has to carry a child for nearly a year before birth is a stern reality. During that period, there are limits to the work that she can perform.

Furthermore, it takes close to twenty years from the time that a child is born until he or she reaches adulthood. There is no other animal species besides the human being, which takes twenty years to reach maturity. Most animals can move right after birth and they reach adulthood within a year. However, it takes twenty years for a human being. Here we have to realize that there is a definite plan at work. A woman's giving birth to a child and then going through the process of raising that child are sacred tasks, and there is a mechanism at work designed to show her just what a momentous undertaking it is.

Nevertheless, there is still room for study as to whether this mechanism is unchangeable or not. Although there could be a different means, it is true that there is a being that created this mechanism thinking, "Human souls can learn more through such a

Part II Chapter 1

Healing Your Mind

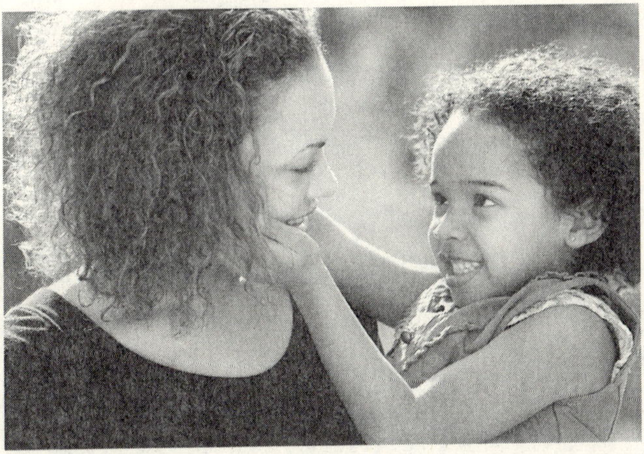

mechanism."

Even though this situation for women might appear to be quite inconvenient, we can find within it the Creator's wish for women to overcome all the distresses and difficulties, including the unstable feelings experienced while undergoing menstruation, and discover that this is the sacred work of maintaining the human species.

If there were no such thing as menstruation, and children just instantly popped out and were born as though they hatched from eggs, it would be easy on the women and their anxiety would no doubt disappear. On the other hand, however, I fear that they would also lose touch with their sacred mission to give life to descendants and then to rear them into adulthood.

Human feelings can waver not just from menstruation, but from illnesses, as well. In fact, very few people become ill without their feelings wavering. Men can also experience mood changes depending upon their physical condition. If a man catches a cold, he will feel weak, but once he recovers, he feels normal.

No one can escape physiological phenomena. To a certain extent, as long as we are living in this world, we cannot escape such physical handicaps. Consequently, what we must do is to adjust our state of mind and concentrate on how to minimize problems and produce better results.

Women may have the handicap of menstruation, but thinking of it as inevitable fate may be looking at menstruation too negatively. I believe that by experiencing feelings of instability, women gain delicateness and elegance, and it is true that they are given the opportunity for introspection. Furthermore, I believe that the fact that a child's soul comes into the physical body of a woman proves that a woman is a far more spiritual existence than a man.

If a man is solely devoting himself to his job, it is likely than he can live a life that has little relationship to spirituality. Yet, since a woman is the "abode of a child," we can say that she is in a sense, a spiritual medium. Since a spirit is lodged in her body for nearly a year, all women can be considered psychics. That is what makes them different from men. Although men do not have to be spiritual, all women by definition have the essential makeup of a psychic.

If you look upon these as "bad facets," then you can no doubt express it as "emotional instability." But if you look upon them as good aspects, they are proof of how the folds of her heart reach deep, how she can understand the feelings of various people, and how she has the capacity to savor such things as art, beauty and literature. I believe that it is important for us to discover these good aspects.

5
Overcoming Past Trauma

Q: What can be done to rid of fears that come from past traumas such as the fear of men due to sexual abuse or obsessive-compulsive neurosis?

A: Psychology has had a lot to say over the past century about sexually related traumas and fears. Nevertheless, as far as I can tell the causes of terror in many cases go beyond experiences in this world—the roots of such fear lie much deeper than that.

Without spiritual readings into past incarnations, we cannot pin down the real cause in any given case. As far as this life is concerned, the causes can vary, including violence experienced when young, or being the victim of sexual abuse and it is not wrong to say, "That is the cause, and that is why you are how you are today." However, deeper investigation in a very great number of cases reveals that the sense of terror can be traced back to former incarnations.

When there is a bitter experience in a past life, such as dying in battle, dying from a major illness, dying from an unexpected accident or being betrayed by another person, the effect of the experience may carry over into this life.

For example, it is only natural that a person who died in a flood will have a fear of water. A person who was killed in a sudden night attack, or an individual who was suddenly and indiscriminately cut down in the street during the era of civil wars, might continuously suffer even in this lifetime from unknown fears. Even though it is possible to find the origin of the fear in this life, the fact is that the root cause is to be found farther in the past.

If in past lives a person was unhappy, and died in unfortunate ways, perhaps perishing in an earthquake,

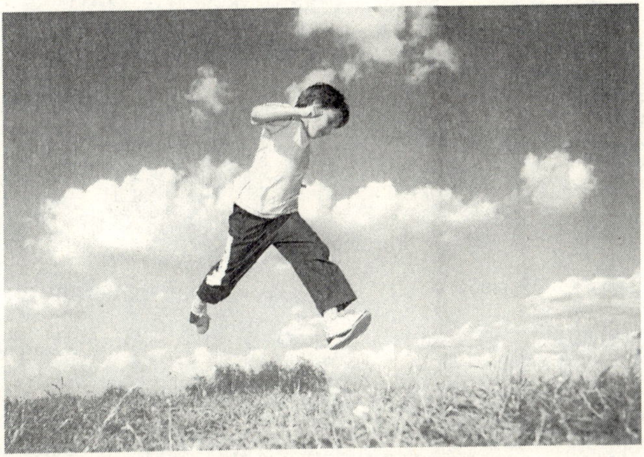

being killed by falling rocks, dying from the plague or having one's village attacked, then the influence of these memories is likely to linger deep within the soul.

Without spiritual investigations, this background will remain totally unknown in this lifetime. However, psychology and other studies are seeking for causes in this lifetime, a shallower place to search.

In the past, I have on numerous occasions taught, "You cannot change the past, but you can change the future. Therefore, work to change the future." Actually, though, there is another step, "If you change the present, then you can even change the past."

The past, as you regard it, is really only "past" as seen through the "eyeglasses of the present." Therefore, if you are happy today, no matter what you may have experienced in the past, everything will seem happy. Can you understand what I am talking about?

Even though you may have experienced various misfortunes long ago such as illness, bankruptcy, lost love, and so forth, if you are happy today, you will think, "Well, by going through all that, I have found my present happiness and all has worked out for the best." In other words, everything will appear as a seed of your present happiness.

However, if you think, "I'm unhappy now," then you will come up with a long list of reasons for your unhappiness: "That illness ruined me," "Failing that test is what did me in," "I'm in this situation because of how she dumped me," "I'm unhappy because our family has gone bankrupt," "I became what I am because my father abused me when I was small," "It's because I was beaten when I was a kid," or, "It's all because my siblings used to kick me around."

Even though people may think that the causes of their unhappiness lie in the past, if right here and now, they choose to be happy, then everything will take on a golden hue. Consequently, the truth is that you can change the past. If you change your present self, your past will also change.

Among people who have achieved great economic success, there are some individuals who will not hesitate to say: "I'm glad that I was poor when I was young. I wanted so badly to escape poverty that I persevered and became what I am today. If my family had been rich, and if I had been affluent, I probably would not have gotten where I am. It was precisely because I was poor that I achieved happiness." Judging from results, that would appear to be the case.

If you are looking for reasons in the past for your present situation, it only goes to show that you are still a bit spoiled. If you allow your present self to give off a shining light, then the past will appear differently.

If you search your past for the reasons you cannot be happy, you will find any numbers of causes. However, everything can also be a "seed of happiness." Exploring your past and discovering the cause that has made you the way you are today, is one method that will give you guidance. Still, the fact is that, if you change yourself right now, then everything in the past will come to appear differently.

The past of this life can change, but you can also consider unhappiness in a past life as the seed for your happiness in this present life. It is true that you can go back that far in time to turn your life around. Please have sufficient fortitude to do just that.

If we can change the past, then changing the future is very simple. Since we are talking about what is going to happen from this point forward, this surely means that there is plenty of room for change.

6

Advice for Those with a Gender Identity Disorder

Q: I have a friend who is suffering from a gender identity disorder. He is perplexed because of the gap between his body and soul, which weighs down on him daily. Please provide some advice for him.

A: Among human beings there are three types: the type that is repeatedly reborn as a man, the type who, like the goddesses, is repeatedly reborn as a female, and the type that takes on both genders. Recently a lot of attention has been paid to people who have a gender identity disorder. This occurs when a person has been born into this life as a man after having been repeatedly born into past lives as a woman, or vice

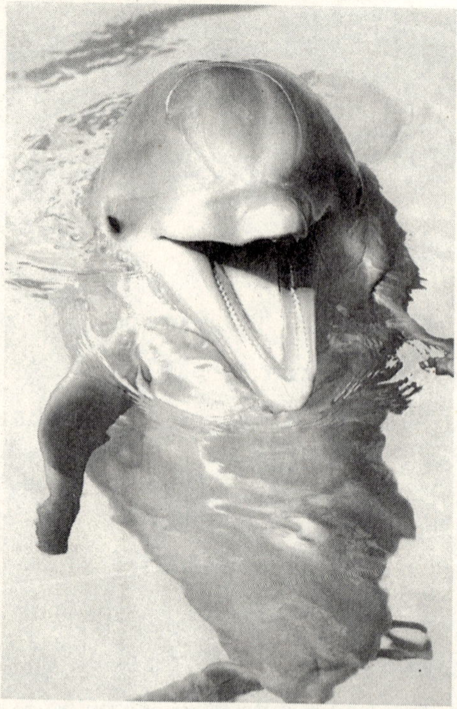

versa. In other words, a person was born as the opposite gender from that of the past, and consequently received a bit of a shock in this case. That is to say, some mistake has been made while the current reincarnation was still in the planning stages.

For example, before the birth was decided a person might have thought, "My parents will absolutely have to be this couple," but it turns out that the pair will only give birth to one child. In such a case, although the intention was to be born as a male, the soul was made to enter into a female body. After birth, the person thinks, "Hey, although I intended to be a man, I ended up being a woman. What a mess I'm in now."

These people did not plan their lives specifically enough. Some people have made perfect plans, others have not. So in the case of individuals with gender identity disorder, the person "miscalculated" and ended up being born in the opposite gender. Nearly all of these people have made this mistake. Consequently, if a person feels strong gender conflictions, it means that his or her soul recognizes the self as the opposite sex.

What happens to a soul's gender when it returns to the other world?

If a person lives as a woman in this world, when she returns to the other world, normally she will retain the consciousness of a woman until she is ready for the next incarnation. Similarly, it is normal for a man to retain a male consciousness. That being so, I think that in your friend's case, his life plan was distorted.

Nowadays, there are cases of intentional abortion and many other complications. An individual may end up marrying someone other than who was intended, or conditions may change a bit so as to throw the predetermined life plan off. In many cases, things may not come off as intended.

However, even if a person is born with the opposite gender from what was intended, if that individual has a mixed-gender group of "soul siblings," he will generally accept the fact. In addition, even if it is the first time for the individual to be born as male or female, the soul may accept the situation and live his or her life.

However, in your friend's case, I think that his soul

cannot accept the situation under any circumstances. Since his soul is oriented to the sex opposite to that of his body, he cannot eliminate the feeling, "This is not me."

In most cases, this kind of situation tends to arise strongly when all the soul siblings are female or male and the individual is born into the opposite sex. However, when the long trail of reincarnations are considered, many are born alternatively as male and female. This is because unless a soul takes on both genders, the life experience is likely to be insufficient.

Although your friend may have been born with the unintended gender this time, it could very well prove a valuable experience for his soul. Therefore, one option is making a go at living with the circumstances. However, if he is determined to stick to his decision of not accepting his current gender, I believe that another option would be gender reassignment surgery.

Since a doctor is unaware that gender identity disorder can be understood in spiritual terms and is not a physical malady, they diagnose it as an illness. Nevertheless, from a religious standpoint, it is not a "disease." It is merely a case of being clearly conscious of one's own sexual nature.

Please inform your friend that this is the basic meaning of the condition. As for how he should live his life, that is up to each individual to decide.

The truth is that if a person lives his whole life with a grudge, he accomplishes nothing. At some point, a person has to make a firm decision. After all, in life we cannot expect everything to go the way we want.

For example, many people are preoccupied with all aspects of their persons: from their height and weight, to how they look, to how smart they are. These people suffer because things are not the way they want them to be. Likewise, there are many people whose reality differs from their pre-birth life plan, and who believe that, "This is not the way things were supposed to be."

Everyone is enduring these complications. Please do not feel isolated and work hard.

7

Abortion from the Spiritual Perspective

Q: You teach, "Human beings are born in accordance with a life plan made in Heaven." But what happens to a soul that is aborted and is therefore unable to be born as scheduled?

A: The problem of abortion (intentional miscarriage) has arisen because almost all human beings are unaware of the mechanism by which souls are reborn.

Because of abortions, Heaven is now in a state of utter confusion. The various spirits of Heaven are troubled. Although they are eager to come to Earth, there are cases in which individuals with important plans are aborted. Even the spirits of Heaven are unable to control the thoughts of people on Earth. Human beings on Earth simply do not act as the spirits of Heaven would like. This is because God endowed human beings with the attribute of subjectivity.

For example, in the section, "Spiritual Conversations with Murasaki Shikibu," from my book, *Ryuho Okawa Collection of Spiritual Messages, Volume 14* (printed by Happy Science, limited to members), Murasaki Shikibu (the famous author of *The Tale of Genji*) declares from Heaven, "Although I was supposed to be reborn in this modern age, because of an abortion, I was not able to do so."

In Murasaki Shikibu's case, because of the clash between the free will of her intended parents on Earth and the free will of Murasaki Shikibu, it turned out that the free will of the people on Earth was stronger.

Because of abortions, the spirit world is currently in great confusion. In Japan today, the reported number of abortions is close to 300,000 cases annually. If those which go unreported are included, it is said that the total climbs to around one million. This will indeed distort the plans for rebirth.

Moreover, although great effort had been taken to lay out life plans for a lifespan of decades and souls were ready to come to this earthly world, since they ended up being aborted while in their mothers' wombs, that fact remains as wounds in these souls. As a result, the next time they consider going to Earth, they are confronted with the fear that the same thing may happen again.

Furthermore, if a soul was born and breathed the air of Earth, or even if it had grown within the womb to the state where it developed the will of a human being, then it has no other choice but to return to Heaven as a soul in the form of an infant, as it cannot immediately regain its previous adult form.

It would take about twenty earthly years for the soul to develop to have an adult consciousness. The spirits that have a connection to this individual will therefore have to care for this spiritual child in the other world from infancy, up until it can return to the former level of adult consciousness. This is a great setback for the evolution of the soul. Abortion should be avoided

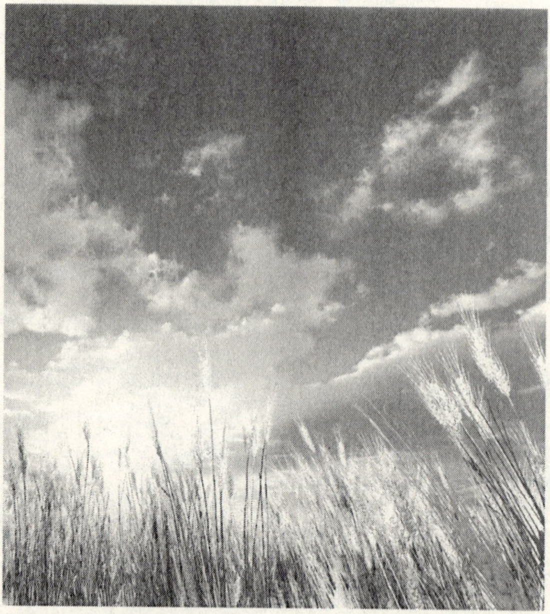

whenever possible.

However, there are times when, because of economic or physical conditions, there is no other alternative. For example, if the mother's body is so weak that childbirth would kill her, it may be unavoidable in order to protect the mother. In such a case, abortion may be acceptable.

In such cases, it is critical that both parents offer sufficient prayers so that the soul which had intended to appear on Earth will be able to mature in the other world without fail and will not continue to feel hurt. I believe that this is their minimum duty as human beings.

Although in principle it is best to avoid abortions, in situations where they become absolute necessities, you must not forget to wish for the happiness of the child's soul, which was unable to be born. However, even while saying that, it is also important not to become attached to it.

AIDS, Influenza, etc.,

With medicine, no matter how much research is done on treatment methods for existing diseases, new diseases continue to appear in rapid succession.

Take AIDS, for instance. Even if a cure were to be found, there is no doubt that a new and different disease would subsequently take its place. Do you know why?

The AIDS virus was discovered during the first half of the 1980s, and quickly became infamous. The fact, though, is that there are spirits at work through this pathogen. These are the same spirits, which in an earlier age spread the plague (Black Death) and cholera. After these diseases had gradually been eliminated thanks to advances in medical science, they slowly transformed themselves and eventually reappeared as AIDS.

If AIDS is suppressed, it will again reappear as still another disease. This is because the spirits are always coming up with new strategies for survival. In this manner, pathogens, too, are influenced by spiritual elements; this cannot be ignored.

In addition, if we look at the situation for colds and influenza, we find that the symptoms they induce bear very strong similarities to spiritual possession. In fact, we can say that the principles involved are very similar to those for possession.

What Spreads a Virus

After meeting someone who has caught a cold and was coughing, your head starts spinning, and not long afterwards you, too, begin to cough–no doubt many people have had such an experience, and in spiritual terms it is an identical phenomenon to spiritual possession. The fact is that spirits cause colds and influenza. Exactly what kind of spirits might they be?

When the weather turns chilly and colds and influenza start spreading, think carefully as to whether there is anything around you at that time which could become a spirit.

Of course there are–insects. When autumn arrives and the weather quickly cools down, insects die off. From around that point, colds and influenza begin to become prevalent. The spirits of some dead insects that cannot return to the other world, become wandering souls, and gather in bands and swarm about through the air. In fact, the spread of colds and influenza is due to these insect souls.

Of course, viruses and bacteria are the pathogens, but they, on their own, are not that harmful. It is only when spiritual manipulation is added that they become much more contagious. In other words, the virus is the kernel on which the insect spirits possess. This is the actual situation.

Don't you find it peculiar? Although viruses themselves are alive in spring and summer, in fact all year round, why should it be that they spread during the winter? The reason is that it is during the winter months that they come under spiritual influence, thus enormously increasing their power.

After that, it is the same as the principle of possession. The process for contagion of colds and influenza is the same as for possession. Here, the swarms of insect souls are exerting their influence. That is the reason why a cold or influenza seems to spread so very rapidly. Many viruses exist but they are not the sole cause.

Hay fever also has spiritual causes. Of course, one cause of hay fever is the pollen of cedar trees. However, the pollen from the trees alone would not be able to cause that much trouble. There is a considerable spiritual influence at work here, also.

Since we continue to build golf courses, etc. and carve up our mountains in various ways, I have the feeling that the assembled spirits of trees and other forms of vegetation which once called these places their homes are also at work to a large extent.

When a disease is rapidly spreading like this, whether it is the plague (Black Death) or cholera, it means that they are all under spiritual influence. If we are not aware of this, I do not believe we will be able to come up with real solutions. Even if we eliminate AIDS, the next disease will take its place. The root source is always the same.

About Various Diseases

1
The Causes of Atopic Dermatitis

Q: My child has eczema. I have tried everything, from taking him to see the doctor to paying careful attention to what I give him to eat, but the eczema is not clearing up.

A: When considering the causes of eczema, it is important to ask yourself what might be wrong in a person's mind that is finding symbolic expression on the skin's surface. You must take into consideration what part of your mind is wrong, that might also be causing afflictions of the skin.

The skin separates the inside of the body from everything outside of it—it acts as a partition between the body and the world around it. Thus, skin abnormalities suggest discontinuity between inside and outside.

"Inside and outside" refer, of course, to the "individual's awareness and soul," and "relationship with others." With children, inside and outside also refer to what is within the home and what is outside of it. In other words, the skin is the borderline between "self" and "others," and also between "inside of the household" and "outside of the household." When there is a problem with this border, then eczema is the result. It comes from a rejection of the outside world.

In addition, the reason that people seek to cut themselves off from everyone and everything else is that they feel what will harm them is outside of them. That is why they react extremely to everything, which is "other."

It follows, then, that if someone in a family has feelings such as these, those feelings might manifest themselves as atopic dermatitis in the children of that family. I think it is highly likely that something or someone in your household may be the cause of your ailments. Please consider this.

It is probably the case that you, or perhaps your spouse or someone else in your family, are causing a strong allergic reaction against those outside of your home. I find it probable that someone has elements, which seek to avoid close relations with other people—some kind of allergic reaction to others. It is important that you resolve that issue. Although it might sound unusual to you, the entirety of the family itself is reflected in that family's children. Children react very sensitively to such things.

Skin problems are a manifestation of some sort of difficulty in your relations with the outside world. This is why you must practice meditation and wish for harmonious relations with others. If it turns out that the cause does not lie with you, then put this meditation exercise into practice as a family.

Naturally, there are other more individualized treatments that you can try, but in a general way of speaking, the above solution is quite plausible.

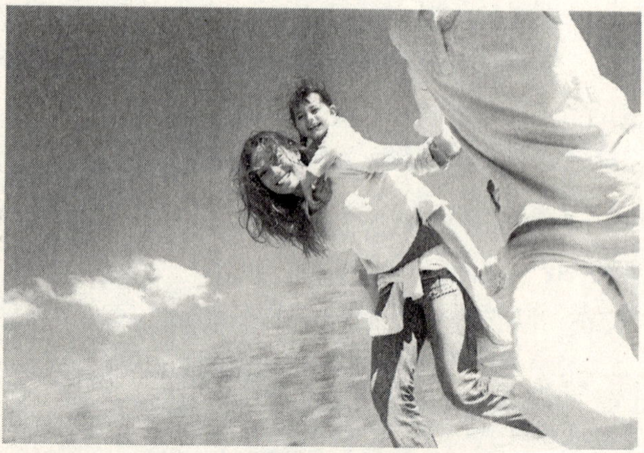

2
The Causes of Autism

Q: Please tell me what causes autism and Asperger syndrome in children, and how I should interact with children afflicted with these conditions.

A: Many scientists classify their research objective into different categories and analyze just about anything under the sun. I have no quarrel with these researchers as such, and think that their approach—their scientific outlook—is not in itself a bad thing.

However, no matter what we might be talking about, when we look at something through colored lenses, then we're going to see everything tinted, and we will believe that the way we see things is really the way things actually are.

If, for example, a physician tells us that someone is autistic, then we find ourselves agreeing with whatever the physician says, and we eventually lose our ability to see any other possibilities than that of the diagnosis. In addition, we often hear that children who are always on the go have been diagnosed as having ADHD, but the fact is that children are active and highly animated by nature.

When a parent takes their child to the doctor's office and is told that their young one has hyperactive disorder, then the parent will forever after think that their child is hyperactive. Yet, if the doctor simply says that the child is reasonably active, the parent will come to agree with that decision, too.

We are told that autism is a disorder and not a disease, but are also told at the same time that autistic people suffer from problems in the functions of the human body. We are told that they have problems in certain areas of the brain. However, this is nothing but an imagination. Doctors have absolutely no idea of what the truth really is.

There are all kinds of different people in this world. Doctors are quick to use the label "autistic" on anyone whose unusual behavior and strange actions are troublesome to deal with and end up causing headaches for parents and teachers. The problem, though, is that this definition of autism is entirely too broad.

It may, indeed, be the case that such children will face difficulties as they try to make their way in a management society. They might have a hard time finding a steady job. This may be correct. When you look more closely, though, you will see that everyone today, who is making a name for oneself, is an unusual person. The easy-to-manage types are suitable to work as underlings, but everyone who starts something original is "strange." Someone even wrote a book titled, *Great Men are All Unusual*. Thomas Edison was unusual, Ryouma Sakamoto was unusual, and I, myself, am unusual.

It is miserable to conform to fixed ways of thinking, which is why I cannot readily accept the things that doctors say. It is especially the case in Japan that whenever anyone is different or has a distinctly individual personality, there is a tendency toward rejection. The Japanese often think that everyone has to be just like everybody else.

However, it is precisely those who have strongly individualistic personalities who go on to change the world. The strong individual is the one who breaks through the status quo and effects unheard-of changes.

If a doctor tells you that your son or daughter is autistic, do not let such a diagnosis trouble you—instead, I would like you to have faith that your child has a strongly individualistic personality. If you think along these lines, then everything will turn out well.

Many of the children whom doctors today label as being autistic will quite possibly go on to make earth-shattering inventions and discoveries, while those children characterized as being hyperactive have every chance of growing up to be explorers.

Doctors put these kinds of labels on children because they cannot take responsibility for what happens after children become adults. These "unusual" children are very often those with the power to change the world. We must give up those old values, which tell us that something is bad just because it is different from everyone else. Do not be so quick to judge your child as being ill or disabled in any way.

Asperger syndrome, a species of autism, is known to be a high-function disorder. Physicians characterize Asperger syndrome patients as having extremely high intelligence, but as being, in a way, autistic.

The fact, though, is that these children are actually geniuses. Many child prodigies are different from everyone else. If we apply the definitions that doctors use, then even Einstein would have to be declared autistic, and to have been suffering from Asperger syndrome. How in the world can we classify such a towering genius as having Asperger syndrome?

Thus, you have to take everything that doctors say with a grain of salt. Do not take doctors seriously when they spout off such phrases as "high-function disability." The characteristics of those with Asperger syndrome overlap in many ways with the features of those who are angels of light. Namely, both are very particular about cleanliness, have strong senses of justice and fairness, and always fight against evil.

If we go by the definitions that doctors have come up with, then everyone who has battled diligently against the forces of evil, and everyone who has brought about religious reforms in the past, was suffering from Asperger syndrome. If we let doctors have their say, then all of these people would be left in obscurity, which would be a shameful thing to have happen.

Angels are very particular in their love of cleanliness, and engage in battle with great forces of evil, which makes them look highly irregular in the eyes of physicians. If we are not careful then doctors will have us convinced that they are all sick. There are many different kinds of people in this world. Human beings can transform through the power of faith, so please supply your child's soul with strength.

3

The Significance of Childhood Disabilities

Q: Some children are stricken with diseases or disabilities at the young age of two or three years old. Are these afflictions a part of the plan for that child's life?

A: Some illnesses are brought about because that person has problems within his or her mind. Nevertheless, when a child of two or three becomes ill, many are apt to think that, surely, someone so young could not possibly have such an evil mind as that. There may be a few differences between the ages of two and three, but all children are apt not to show such profound changes between these two ages.

There are general theories and individual theories to explain the issue of children who become sick.

The general theories go something like this:

Small children reflect the situation of the household in which they live. Because the child's parents are closest to the child, the state of the parents' minds is manifested directly in the child. Children, who have not yet developed a sense of "self" as adults have, are highly influenced by their parents.

For this reason, we should look to the parents, and not the children. If a child becomes sick, it is most likely that there is something wrong in the mind of the child's parents. Then, that manifests in the physical condition of the child. Many phenomena arise because of the state of mind. Whenever a child falls ill, it is generally the case that the child's parents or someone close to the child has some kind of problem.

If we look at this as an individual issue, we can understand that it is not necessarily the case that the problem lies with the parents or other people who play a major role in a child's life. The basis for this way of thinking lies in the examples offered by people such as Helen Keller.

A disease during childhood left Helen Keller blind and deaf. If she had not been so cruelly stricken, though—if she had gone through life in a normal body—then she would have been considered to be nothing more than a talented woman, regardless of how wonderful her writings may have been. As a sighted and hearing person, she would not have been able to inspire the world with such courage and bravery as she did.

It is precisely because she triumphed over such harsh handicaps that she was able to cast forth a light of hope for many people with disabilities. If someone who enjoyed full use of limbs and senses were to tell us that we must learn to be satisfied even if we were blind and deaf, there are many among us who would reject these words. However, the voice of someone who has come to shine with inner light through experience is very strong.

In Chapter 2 of, *Ryuho Okawa Collection of Spiritual Messages, Vol. 17*, (printed by Happy Science, limited to members), this is discussed as the "Principles of

Conversion" by the spirit of Yuien (1222-1289), a disciple of Shinran (1173-1262) and the author of *Tannishou* (*Lamentations of Divergences*). According to Yuien, high spirits sometimes create a situation where a truly evil person will right himself completely, thus affording those in a similar state the opportunity to reverse the course of their lives, as well.

Many people resist accepting the message of one who is born a saint or a gentleman, when he preaches the way. These people say, "It's easy enough for you to speak of such things, living as you do like a fine fish in clear water, but someone from a transparent stream could never understand the way of those who live down in the muddy gutter water."

It is for saving these wretched souls that, at a certain rate, truly evil persons will return to the path of righteousness.

In America around the turn of the twentieth century, the boss of a gang of armed robbers rose up out of the ashes of his many sins and began to preach the word of God under the name of Starr Daily. Other people looked upon him and were given hope, because if someone like him could cast off his sins and rise again to do the work of God, then surely any other street urchin could do the same. This is one of the tactics employed by the high spirits.

For instance, despite being told that you have heart disease, if you do not resign yourself to unhappiness but instead go on to do great things, you could shine the light of salvation for others. It is for this reason that great men and women are sometimes made to live with disabilities. Thus, some people are intentionally born with severe handicaps so that they may serve as a model for other people.

During the Showa Era (1926-1989), there was a genius painter with a mental handicap called, Kiyoshi Yamashita (1922-1951) who was famous for his masterly works in collage. This man was a high spirit from the realm of the bodhisattvas. An angel of light descended to earth in the form of a mentally retarded man in order to give courage to others suffering from handicaps.

People from the other world might find it pitiful that

an angel of light should take on the form of someone with a mental disorder, but this was done for the sake of a much bigger purpose. Human beings on earth cannot comprehend this, but the point of this man's existence was to provide a model of an exemplary life lived to the fullest despite having to bear the burden of being handicapped.

Ultimately, then, to answer your question, I would say that a person's life is a workbook of problems to be solved.

In a general sense, when a child is beset by illness, the state of mind of the child's parents and other close people is reflected in that child's health, but there are also other, more individual reasons that a child might become sick. Even those destined for greatness might fall ill. In addition, the reason for it is to show people that there are many different ways in which a person might live out his or her life.

Therefore, if you happen to be handicapped in some way, I would like you to press ahead resolutely in the belief that you, too, have a special mission to fulfill.

4
Overcoming Stuttering

Q: I tend to get agitated easily and although I do not usually stammer, whenever I have to speak in front of a group of people, or whenever there is a crowd watching me while I speak, I end up stuttering. Please teach me a good way to overcome this speech impediment.

A: Approximately seventy to eighty percent of all cases of stuttering problems come from a spiritual cause. When someone who stutters passes away and his or her spirit possesses another living person, then the possessed person also begins to stutter.

The treatment in such a case is the same as with any

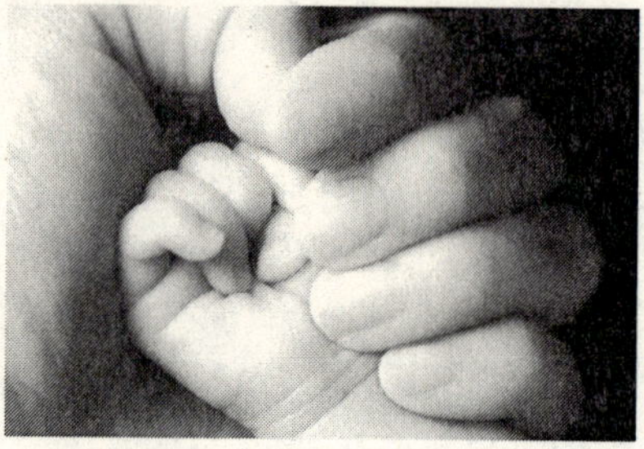

other way of ridding possessing spirits. It is important to clear away the clouds that cover the mind and to strengthen the amount of light within.

The next is a treatment method for stuttering caused by non-spiritual factors. Stuttering can often readily be overcome through training and practice.

People who stutter tend to be timid, retiring and cowardly. Thus, whenever they are made to stand up and talk in front of people, they over-react to the situation. It all comes down to the fact that these people feel a deep sense of inferiority. There is no doubt about it. They have a very negative image of who they are. They are overwhelmingly ashamed of who they are, so they become embarrassed whenever someone sees them or hears them speak. They want to hide away and avoid being exposed to the harsh gaze of other people. Then it becomes a struggle with these negative feelings. Can someone overcome these emotions, or can't they—that is the question at hand.

It also frequently happens that those who are poor at giving speeches are the same people who have nothing to talk about. They think of themselves as having nothing about which they are qualified to hold forth, so they slink into the corner.

One way to overcome these feelings is to find and learn something you can talk about without being embarrassed. If you become expert in a certain field, you may be surprised to find that you actually want to go out and speak to people about it.

Another method to try is to make a full effort to study the area that you are most unsure of. It is said that fear will follow us no matter how much we try to flee from it. The more you are afraid of something, the more it will come after you. Thus, if you are trying to overcome a stuttering problem, the only thing to do is to put yourself in a position in which you will be forced to give a public speech.

This is an extremely important point. Even if you are a very delicate type of person, as you gain experience you will also increase your stock of courage, and gradually your mind will become less wavering. With experience, you will become more daring, and will think of it as nothing at all to stand up in front of people and deliver a speech—you simply will not care what the folks in your audience might think about you.

Moreover, when you get to that point, there is nothing more to worry. You are overly conscious of what others think when they look at you, which is why you get flustered and begin to stutter—the best remedy for this is to become unconcerned with everyone else's opinions. In addition, the best way to achieve this is through the accumulation of experience.

For this, you should be proactive in creating some situation for you to stand up before others and speak. It is important for you to set your mind on speaking in front of people.

Where there is a will, there is a way.

5
Treatments for Rheumatism

Q: My daughter has rheumatism, and is bed-ridden throughout most of the day. Please tell me what causes rheumatism, and what I can do to help her get better.

A: Rheumatism is almost exclusively caused by spiritual possession. It is common that animal spirits (originally humans) have taken possession of the lower halves of bodies, but when these spirits become completely stuck to us, then we experience chronic chills in the lower body, and our bodies become unable to move. There are also cases, of course, in which these spirits possess us in our shoulders and necks.

It is most certain that such a spirit also possesses your daughter.

If the patient herself cannot practice self-reflection or move, then there's no other option but for those around her to make efforts. The other family members must correct their minds, and must strengthen the light that they emit. I believe that by doing so the possessing

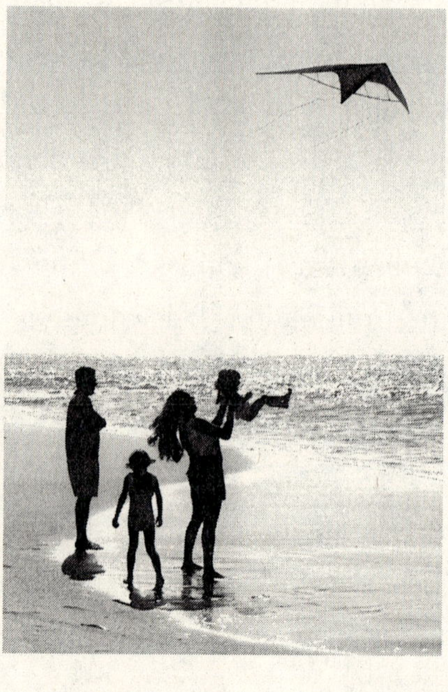

spirit will come off your daughter's body.

If it is a possessing spirit, then in a certain sense this makes the illness easy to heal—if the spirit, that causes an illness, can be expelled, then the patient will make a full recovery. This method will derive one hundred percent effect.

I think that as the parent of the girl who is afflicted, you must have a certain degree of understanding regarding what might have brought her to such a pass. When you examine the life that your daughter has led under the light of the Truth, can you find any mistakes she has made? If not, then perhaps your daughter has come under some sort of negative influence from other family members or others with whom she associates. Please think about the problem along these lines.

Some people are spiritually sensitive and they keenly sense the existence of spirits. Evil spirits that have been attached to someone nearby, even though they might not have done anything particularly bad to cause such a possession, sometimes possess such people. Evil spirits always seek out the person in the family who is the weakest, and who is thus the easiest prey.

First, examine the person herself and see if there is any fault to be found with her. If not, then ask yourself if there is anyone else in the family who might be leading a life with mistaken thoughts or feelings. If such a person is found, they must start reflecting on themselves.

If that person is incapable of reflecting upon his or her own actions, then the people around that person must first provide an example to follow. The other members of the family must strengthen the light they emit, and strive to create a close-knit, warm and lively household. You must not make a cold and indifferent home or in which all of the family members blame one another for everything that goes wrong.

You and your other family members must have courage, shine forth a stronger light, and wish to heal your daughter's sickness. I have complete faith that she is going to get better.

6
The Spiritual Significance of Incurable Diseases

Q: I am a medical student undergoing clinical training at a hospital; there are many young patients there who are suffering from leukemia and other incurable diseases. Please teach me the causes of incurable diseases, and the spiritual significance that such diseases might have.

A: First, when we speak of leukemia and other blood-related diseases, we must say that these kinds of afflictions are clearly caused by spiritual factors.

What is it, though, that could affect the bloodstream? A person's blood is the very source of life; it is what nourishes one's being. It is often the case that a person suffering from a blood disease has within him an element within that is obstructing the development and prosperity of that person's life.

There are two kinds of elements, which stand in obstruction of the development and prosperity of life.

The first such element is the karma that was engraved into the soul before it was born on earth (see p. 72, "The Truth about Mind and Body 2"). Sadly enough, while it pains me to say so, people, who in a former life brought harm to the lives of others, and thus have such karma, are more likely to come down with blood-related illnesses.

In more concrete terms, if someone, in a past life, spilled the blood of someone else or participated in some kind of event in which the lives of other people were taken away, then the soul has a memory of this scene, and it is engraved deeply within.

If this soul goes to the world beyond ours—that is, to the afterlife—and completely resolves all sins, then the matter will end there. However, usually, it cannot be perfectly cleared in the other world. So in many cases, the souls are reborn on earth for continuing to resolve the karma.

The soul wishes to clear up the mistaken thoughts and actions, and so descends back to this world with that plan. When such people are reborn, then the karma often materializes as blood-related ailments. These kinds of illnesses might not appear during childhood but they will gradually manifest later in the person's adult life.

These kinds of people have souls that long for self-destruction. They spilled blood in a past life, and now wish to torture themselves for it. It is this thinking that could be giving rise to the pathological phenomena.

You might think that human beings are crafted out of nature, but the truth is that the will shapes the body and maintains it. If, in the will, there are unnoticed feelings of self-punishment in the subconscious, then it becomes quite easy for pathological phenomena to occur. In a sense, these people are the ones that will find it hard to avoid the illnesses.

Evil spirits are another element obstructing the development and prosperity of life. When an evil spirit possesses you, sometimes you develop symptoms identical to the disease that killed the spirit.

If, for example, you are possessed by the wandering spirit of someone who died of a blood-related illness such as those associated with radiation poisoning incurred from an atomic blast, then you yourself will come down with a similar sickness. This is because the will of human beings has the power to materialize things.

Almost all of the pathological phenomena, which afflict the body, form in this way. Even though you possess within yourself the power to eliminate these evil substances, when you are influenced spiritually, then this power you have is weakened, and evil takes root and flourishes.

There are many strange and incurable diseases today, but there are also a great number of new diseases making an appearance. A disease is a manifestation of a thought with a certain vector. Whenever your thinking inclines towards a certain direction, this appears in your body. Thus, when the taking of pills and medical attention blocks the exit points of these ways of thinking, they find new places from which to appear.

One case in point: when the plague and cholera which once beset mankind was eradicated, they reappeared again in the form of new diseases such as AIDS (see p. 118, "The Truth about Mind and Body 3").

When the "thought cloud of disease," the conception of the disease itself, is prevented in some kind of way, it will find another route and take shape as something else. Strangely enough, there are now an extraordinarily large number of cases of strange and incurable dermatological diseases. However, why?

There are many animals, mainly in the oceans and rivers, which have been driven out of their habitats by the advancement of highly developed modern metropolitan societies. When pollution destroys their ecosystems and deprives them of a place to live, what happens to these animals?

Fish and other animals all possess the same capacity

for joy, anger, sadness and enjoyment that humans do. This means that they have a sense of happiness and unhappiness, as well. Thus, when their companions' lives are taken en masse for no apparent reason, as a whole, they feel anger and have resentment towards the situation.

For example, there are creatures that have been driven out of rivers because humans have polluted it. These animals suffered greatly before dying. The same thing happened along coastal industrial zones.

Thereafter, the people who live along these waterways may begin to develop ichthyosis, a disease in which the skin takes on a scaly, fish-like appearance. These kinds of diseases can almost never be cured at a hospital, because they are caused by the concentrated resentment and anger of dead animals.

Let us also consider the disease known as muscle atrophy. This disease can also be categorized according to two different causes. The first cause is influence from a past life.

Where does this karma, which causes someone's

muscles to gradually lose their power to flex and move, come from? I think you will all be able to guess—such karma is produced as a reaction to when someone causes someone else to lose freedom of motion.

When we actually look at the past lives of people who have been diagnosed with muscle atrophy, we will find that many of them once deprived others of the ability to freely move their bodies. This kind of thing happens frequently during the chaos of war. If someone takes a defeated prisoner of war into custody and subjects him to hard labor and corporal punishment, then this person may develop muscle atrophy or some other kind of disease in their next life which will limit their ability to move their bodies. This is one aspect of the situation.

The other cause to be considered is, of course, spiritual influence. Animal related spirits are often the culprits in these cases; they possess the arms and legs and through that influence, the patient develops the illness.

Naturally, not everything can be attributed to karma.

There are also those who, like Helen Keller—have endured the double handicap of being deaf and blind—who intentionally choose to be reborn with a handicap for a holy purpose.

Stephen Hawking, the world-famous genius physicist who has muscle atrophy, amyotrophic lateral sclerosis (ALS), is another example of someone who is trying to teach the world something through his disability. There are cases in which someone has taken on a disease as the work of a bodhisattva.

Some people are socially very active despite being confined to a wheelchair. These people might think to themselves, "Why me?" but among them are some that have planned such a destiny, daring to take on the challenge.

It is for the reason of inspiring others with courage, joy and a sense of life's purpose that they have chosen to be born with a physical disability. When seen in a spiritual sense, these kinds of sufferings are over in the blink of an eye. Some people choose to live such a life with the objective of obtaining the virtue that suffering

Part II Chapter 2

About Various Diseases

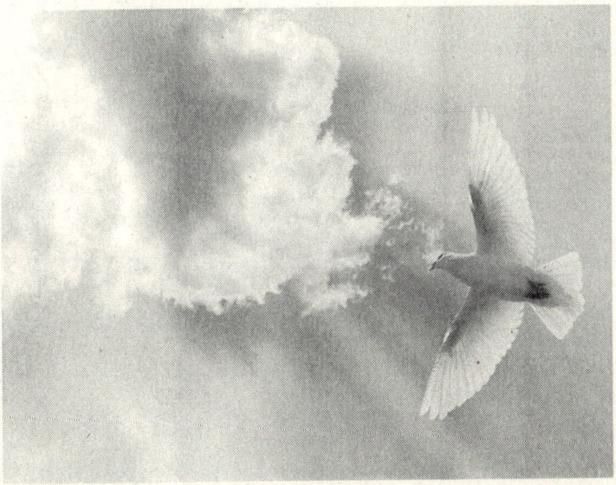

affords. When they leave this world, all of their physical disabilities evaporate, and they regain the freedom that they once had.

While I cannot speak definitively for every single patient, I can nevertheless say that in a broad sense strange and incurable diseases can possibly be divided into the three categories that I have been outlining above. Either these patients have created the causes of their diseases in a previous life, or they have fallen ill due to influence from evil spirits. They could have also intentionally chosen their disability as part of their mission.

One of these three things should explain the illnesses that these patients face, but according to the principle of self-responsibility, most people will fall into the first or the second set.

If the patient is from the second group—those who are affected by evil spirits—then the problem lies in the mind. As I have written repeatedly in my books, there is a principle known as the "Law of the Same Wavelengths' Attraction"—your mind becomes connected to the realms that have the same wavelengths as the wavelengths that your mind sends out.

It follows, then, that if someone is receiving evil spiritual wavelengths, the cause of this unwelcome reception is with the person. Please be aware, though, that even if we say that the cause lies with the patient, there is an enormous amount of variation within this seemingly simple explanation.

It could very well be, for instance, that the troubles of family members are the cause of the problem, but in any event, the patient is the one who has actually received and took the poison. Unless that intake is cleared away, the spiritual influence cannot be cut off.

According to the Law of the "Same Wavelengths' Attraction," if your wavelengths do not match those of evil spirits, then those spirits will not come to you, which is why you must tune your heart to a completely different channel. The wavelength you should set your dial to is that of the high spirits.

In order to find the wavelength of the high spirits, you should think bright and positive thoughts, and should fill your heart to overflowing with hope, love and courage. In other words, abandon your negative thoughts, turn your mind towards an assertive direction and choose to live your life in a positive way.

I also expect that if the family of someone suffering from a disease makes an effort to live in such a positive manner, this will brighten up the entire household, as well. Seventy or eighty percent of diseases are caused almost exclusively by one's state of mind. Firstly, it is important to realize that there is something within you that is calling in the illness, and start by correcting that part.

7
A Guide for Those who Have Lost Their Sight

Q: I have lost the use of my eyes, although I was once sighted. What sort of mindset should I maintain as I make my way through life?

A: Everyone has different sufferings. You have your own sufferings, and when you consider my position you might think it enviable to be me, but I, too, have my own sufferings.

People are prone to think that everyone else is happy and that they alone have been given a heavy cross to carry. When they see things in this way, it is easy for them to look at others and feel that the handicap that they themselves have is the cause of their unhappiness.

"Oh, if only I could rid of this affliction, then I could be happy just like everybody else!"

However, it is unadvisable to assume that whenever there is a marked difference between you and other people in terms of environment, character, physical endowments or overall ability, that this is nothing but a cause for suffering, and then to seek a way out of the situation.

Actually, within the sources of your worry and concern, which everyone recognizes, you may be able to find the key to solving the workbook of problems presented to you by your life. I would like you to bear this in mind.

The fact that you are blind is something, which will bring about progress for your soul. You might not be able to understand its significance in this life, but by living your life within a body that has been handicapped, I think that you feel very keenly that to have full use of one's limbs is something about which a person can be extraordinarily happy.

We often hear the expression, "I never knew what a

blessing health was until the first time I became sick." Some people who have free use of their arms and legs, and who can see and hear, never realize just how lucky they are.

There are many people who cannot use their legs, or have no arms, or are blind or deaf, or are stricken with some other physical disability which restricts the freedom of their bodies. Some of these people have karma from their past lives which has caused their disability in the present.

In your particular case, it was necessary for your soul to learn how blessed it is to be able to enjoy sight.

If I do spiritual readings on someone, I am able to follow the thread of their rebirths through countless lives across five thousand or ten thousand years, but going through each of those lives would be a never-ending task.

No matter what happened in our past lives, we must embrace the set of problems handed to us in our present life, and make an effort to find the answers to those problems and questions. This workbook of problems to

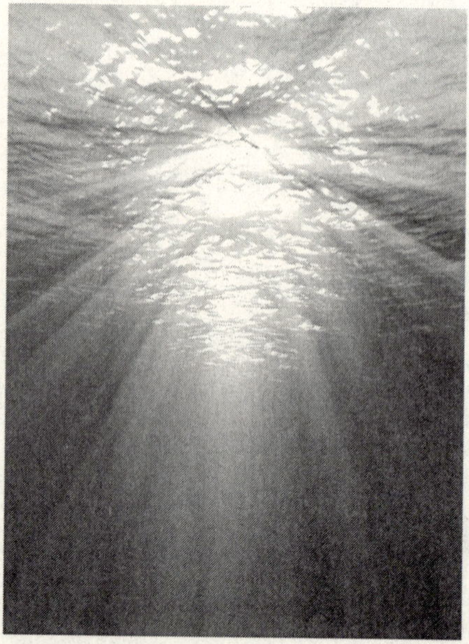

be solved is different for each person. The only fact is that the workbook will be perfectly suited to the study that each individual's soul must undertake.

We must not flee from our problems, nor must we avoid the work of finding the solutions that those problems call for. I would like for all of you to seek out the significance that is hidden within the problems that you face.

You may be blind, but I would like you to find some way to live a shining life in spite of your handicap. Your life can be considered a success if others who enjoy good eyesight look at you and say to themselves, "If someone who cannot see has nevertheless become such a splendid person, then I must certainly make more efforts than I have been."

Physical handicaps disappear when you return to the other world. Blindness and deafness are made right again, when you go on to the next world. Our disabilities last only so long as our time here on earth does, which equals the span of merely a few decades. This is the truth.

The role into which you have been cast in this life is a part of your ongoing spiritual development. Do not become fixated on the thought that if only your physical disabilities were cured you would then be able to become happy. Instead, you must seek to live the best life you possibly can within the circumstances in which you placed yourself in this life. You may burden others as you move forward towards your own best self, but there will also be things you can give in return. Therefore, I would like you to make efforts to think less of the negative and to focus only on the positive in everything that you do.

Your physical eyes may not allow you to see, but the eye of your mind can never be darkened. There is nothing preventing you from finding the Truth with an inner sight that no one can take away from you. From there, you will be able to produce something positive through speaking or listening or any of the other faculties and senses which remain with you.

This is all a part of the "workbook of problems," which has been assigned to you. It is up to you to work to solve these problems now, in this lifetime, and with your own steam. The answers to the problems in this workbook will be handed to you when you return to the other world. You will come to understand then, why you were made to undergo the specific spiritual training that you are now carrying out. Until that day comes, devote yourself wholeheartedly to solving the set of problems that have been given to you.

Buddhism and Longevity

Years and decades of sustained profound contemplative activities will lead to longer life. When people of religion become lazy in their studies and spiritual practices and run out of things to say, they quickly wither and die.

Shinran, for instance, enjoyed full mental capacity even at the age of ninety. The reason for his undiminished mental faculty was Shinran's complete devotion to two decades of study when he was younger. This deep well of knowledge allowed him to keep going for as long as he did.

Some people who study Shinran's teachings feel that it is unnecessary to study or to read the scriptures because Shinran says so, but Shinran himself was an avid student.

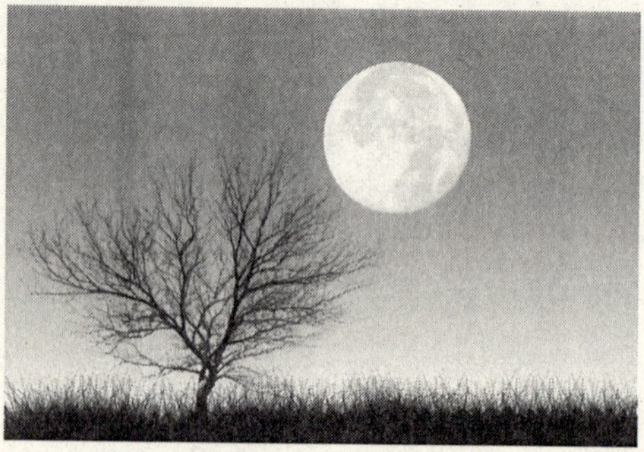

Here was a man who spent twenty years on Mt. Hiei poring through his religious books.

It all starts from the fact that there are many gateways to Shakyamuni Buddha's teachings–in fact, his teachings have 84,000 of these "Dharma gates." It takes a very long time to expound upon all of these different teachings, which is why Shakyamuni Buddha himself had no choice but to live for as long as he did.

On the other hand, because Jesus taught in a very fervent manner, he would not have been able to go on with his ministry for a great length of time. Jesus' teachings were impassioned teachings that would not have allowed him to die of old age.

Theologians and other religious scholars who study Buddhism and Indian philosophy are said to have died "prematurely" if they pass away at the age of seventy or eighty years old. Indian philosophy laments the passing of an eighty-year-old man because he was "still so young." It is the norm for these scholars to live well into their nineties.

One reason for this is that there is so much to study. There are so many sutras in Buddhism that there can never be any end to the study of them, no matter how many years one devotes to the subject. If you are studying the Tripitaka, then you should understand that you will never come to the end of your studies.

One more reason for this longevity is that Buddhism's message is one of serenity and peace. The daily quest to live an ordered life, including reading of sutras, will naturally lead to a very placid temperament. You become peaceful, patient, and very slow to anger, all of which will allow you to live for ninety or more years.

The teachings of Happy Science are also voluminous, but a deep library of teachings is a very good thing. It means that you will be able to live a long life. Please bear this in mind.

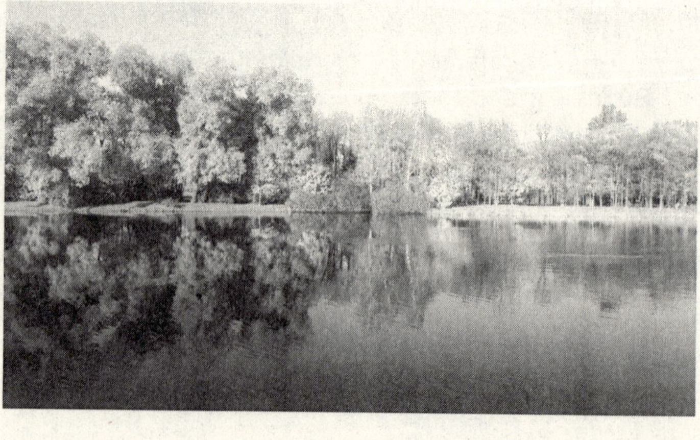

Part II Chapter 3

For Nurses and Caregivers

1

Caring for the Sick

Q: What sort of mindset would be best for me to have when I am caring for people who have fallen ill and are worried?

A: People who are called upon to look after the sick must turn their attention to the words that they use.

Doctors are always made to take responsibility for whatever happens to their patients, so doctors usually offer patients a worst-case scenario diagnosis. If a doctor tells a patient's family that the person is going to make a recovery, only to find that the patient in fact dies, then the doctor will be held liable for it, which is why the doctor always says that things don't look very good. When operating on a patient, the doctor or surgeon will declare that the chances of survival run about fifty-fifty; "I can't guarantee that he'll come out of this alive, but I'm willing to operate on him if he would like to take the chance."

Every doctor has undoubtedly experienced a situation in which he has assured a patient of a full recovery only to witness an unexpected downturn in the patient's condition, which causes doctors to gradually think negatively about patients thereafter.

Words, though, have a power of their own. Those who are caregivers for sick people must offer these patients positive words. If a doctor tells a patient that they are knocking on death's door, then the patient may actually not be able to live long. In addition, if the family is told that the patient has only three months left to live, then everyone begins to believe it and the words become a reality.

On the other hand, though, there are an untold number of cases in which a person who has slipped into despair will suddenly regain his high color, and feel better again after hearing just a single word of encouragement from someone around him. Caregivers for the sick must train themselves to accept nothing less than a full recovery for their charges.

If I were to be hired by a hospital, for instance, there would be a sudden and precipitous drop in the number of patients. I have no medical training whatsoever—simply by making the rounds to the rooms and speaking with the patients, I think they would all come to feel much better and be able to go home. This is what I mean.

Human beings are not physical creatures—they are spiritual beings. The human body is strongly influenced by the mind. Thus, when we are filled with life energy, illnesses are cured.

Human bodies are filled with the natural power of self-healing. When our minds, though, are inclined towards evil and creating sickness, then that is inevitably the direction in which our bodies will proceed.

An analysis of the minds of sick people reveals that not one of them is in harmony with the Truth. These people's minds are filled with complaints, dissatisfaction, jealousy, resentment, grudges, and thoughts of blame for their surroundings and other people. The truth is that a mind filled with such things will make the body sicker than it already is.

By changing these people's minds their bodies also are made right, so, as a caregiver to the sick, I ask you to bear these points in mind as you come into contact with those who are ill.

2

Caring for the Senile

Q: I am currently caring for my mother, who is suffering from dementia and who will soon turn eighty-two. Please tell me how I can best go about interacting with her.

A: At your mother's age, it is not at all surprising that she should be suffering from senility and dementia.

Just because a person has become senile does not mean he or she cannot enter the heavenly world. It is likely that some sort of damage has been done to your mother's brain, and she cannot precisely convey the thoughts of her soul to her body, thus unable to move about, as she would like.

My father, who passed away at the age of eighty-two, had a tumor in a part of his brain and thus was unable to interact freely for about seven months before he died. When he passed away, though, he wrote a haiku poem a day or two after dying and sent spiritual messages to me. The poem can be found in the book, *Saburo Yoshikawa's Spiritual Messages: Sermons after Returning to Heaven 1* (Ryuho Okawa, Printed by Happy Science).

Thus, we can see that even if the brain—the "mechanism" that allows our bodies to move—sustains an injury and our bodies are unable to perform their usual range of motions, our souls remain unharmed. Our souls are normal and in their original state.

My father's soul became younger after death; one or two months after he passed away, his soul was already around sixty-five years old, and then the years continued to fall away, until he returned to his forties.

In this way, the soul is intact, so there is nothing to worry about even in your mother's case. The final days of her life may be a little painful to her, but the suffering she might experience before death will turn into an overwhelming sense of liberation when she passes over to the next world, and will eventually give way to a deep feeling of happiness.

When you care for an elderly person, you are likely to hear all manner of complaints: "My legs won't move. I cannot get out of bed. I am in excruciating pain because of the cancer. Everything hurts. My mind is unclear; I cannot get my thoughts across. My mind is fine, but everyone around me is treating me like I'm crazy..." Everyone experiences restrictions on their freedom when they become old.

However, when we pass on to the next world, we feel like the cicada, which has sprouted wings. We feel light, free, and happy. People bound for Heaven will feel happiness after they have died. People destined for Hell are different from this, but those going to Heaven will feel happy after death.

Your mother, who has dementia, is likely causing you and your family to experience inconvenience on her behalf, and is most likely suffering herself. I believe

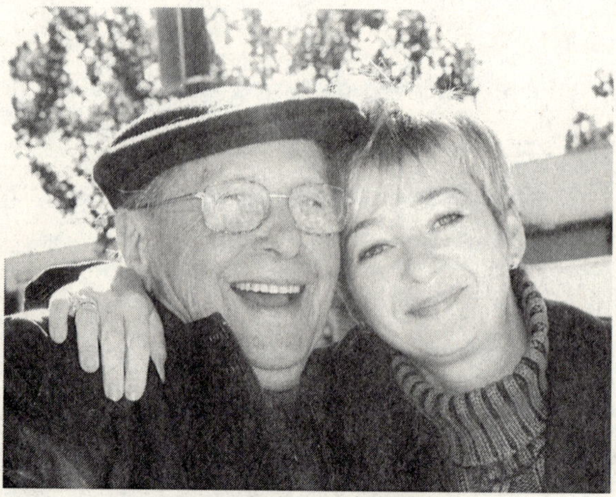

that your mother is apologizing to everyone around her from within her own heart.

It is undoubtedly a difficult time for you and the rest of your family, but the happiness awaiting your mother in the next life will be extremely strong.

Families that take care of the elderly might have a sense of obligation of giving returns or they might be thinking that they themselves will also be taken care of someday; either way, it is a practice of love. Perseverance is also a practice of love.

Furthermore, if someone is afflicted with Alzheimer's disease in his or her later years, this is in no way an indication that that person has led a mistaken life. Just like any other machine, the human body will weaken with age—the brain and the other organs will lose their ability to function properly. Even though the body might weaken, the soul is perfectly well. It is for this reason that you should watch what you say, because there is a high possibility that the person's soul can understand every word that you utter.

I feel that the day is already fixed when your mother

will be "welcomed home," so until that time comes I feel that your family is given the ground to develop its love by putting it into practice toward your mother.

There is nothing to worry about—defects of the flesh have absolutely nothing to do with your mother's ability to ascend into the heavenly world.

3
Overwhelmed with Nursing

Q: One year ago, my husband's mother fell ill and is now confined to her bed almost all day. Between raising the kids, taking care of the household chores and caring for my mother-in-law, I am physically and mentally exhausted. If you have any advice, I would be very happy to hear it.

A: If you look at the big picture, there is almost no one who will never experience having a sick person in his or her household. Sickness, accidents, unforeseen disasters, and the death that comes from these—such events are an occasional part of life. When they occur, they can throw us into a deep pool of sadness.

A home that is spending all day and night caring for the afflicted person must be quite gloomy. However, I believe that you should be careful to avoid looking at only the dark side of your situation.

A human being is, essentially, a soul lodged within a physical body and undergoing spiritual discipline. Even if the body should be affected by disease and suffering, when the soul returns to the other world, it will restore to its original state. The suffering of disease is nothing more than a part of the spiritual discipline within which the soul is engaged here on earth—this suffering will not last forever. No matter how much it might seem that someone is trapped within a Hell of suffering, when their soul leaves their body, it will enter the state of perfect freedom.

As such, what happens after death is far, far more important than the suffering that comes when someone falls ill and is unable to recover. This is because this world is nothing more than a preparatory session in which we practice in order to return to the world beyond. Therefore, no matter what problems you might face, it is vital that you think of those happenings and events as a positive role in the training of your soul. It is best if both sides of the equation—the caregiver and the one who is cared for—look at things in this way.

It is not my intention to say anything cruel to someone who is worn out from looking after a sick person. Still it is within this difficult situation of having a sick person in the home that you are tested as to how warmly, cheerfully and hopefully, you are able to carry on, and therefore allow your soul to shine.

If you look upon sadness and suffering as a rasp for polishing your soul to shine, then you will be able to endure anything, no matter how much pain it might cause you.

Not only this, but it is precisely those times of sadness in which you are offered the opportunity to make rapid religious progress. When times are difficult, people seek salvation and gain a higher level of awareness about your soul.

Do not use the existence of a sick family member as

an excuse not to be happy. Instead, it is important to be grateful for the opportunity to allow your soul to undergo spiritual discipline, and to set your own heart to shining by polishing it against the roughness of your circumstances.

When someone in your household falls ill, it causes you to think about what giving, self-sacrificing, serving love really is, which I believe makes it an opportunity for you to learn what it means to have a heart dedicated to someone else. It is easy to love someone when everything is going well—for example, when your husband is healthy or your wife is beautiful—but when your husband loses his job or your wife's beauty begins to fade, love becomes a much more difficult practice. The heart filled with endurance and tolerance that resolves to love someone in spite of their flaws and shortcomings, though, is the heart that makes love true.

The same holds true with those who are sick. When misfortune befalls someone in our family, with whom we have always gotten along very well, it is then important for us to patiently watch over them. The sick people must also not lament their fate of having fallen ill, but should consider deeply about having to accept the love that other people offer. They should wish to attain peace of mind as soon as possible so they can make things easier for the people around them and bring happiness to those people. You must free yourself from resentment, maintain a serene mind, and devote all of your efforts to curing the sickness you face.

If your luck does not change and you are destined to pass over to the other world, then as long as you were able to keep up the fight against your illness in the laudable frame of mind I suggested above, when you leave your physical body, you will definitely be able to enter the brilliant world of Heaven.

Never hold a grudge against your fate. Take all that comes as nourishment for your soul, and watch as true happiness begins to shine forth.

Improve Your Daily Habits

Many Japanese people die of heart disease, but almost all of these cases are actually caused by daily habits. Heart disease tends to occur when an individual habitually eats fatty or high calorie foods and does not exercise sufficiently.

It means, of course, that heart disease is preventable. Unlike spiritual influences, heart disease is rooted in bodily factors, which means that by looking at the habits people practice in their daily lives, we can tell who will fall ill. If you feel that progressing along your current path will lead to death from heart disease, then the important thing is to make improvements through the power of your will.

When you sit down to eat, it is clear that you should limit your intake of fatty and high-calorie foods. Alcoholic drinks are also loaded with calories, so if you are a heavy drinker then it's imperative that you cut back.

Some businessmen go out drinking at night and gorge themselves on the pretzels and peanuts that they get with their drinks down at the local watering hole. When they finally stumble home, they have a light meal and then turn in. These people probably pay no attention to how much they drink, thinking that alcohol is just like water, but alcohol is very high in calories–it's nothing to ingest three or four thousand calories without even realizing it, which will damage the body if it is kept up for an extended period of time.

and Prevent Heart Disease

Because heart disease is caused by our daily habits, we must start making efforts while we are in our thirties to prevent the disease from developing. Aging begins in our thirties, so we must be proactive in getting an appropriate amount of exercise, eating nutritious foods, maintaining a target weight, and getting enough rest.

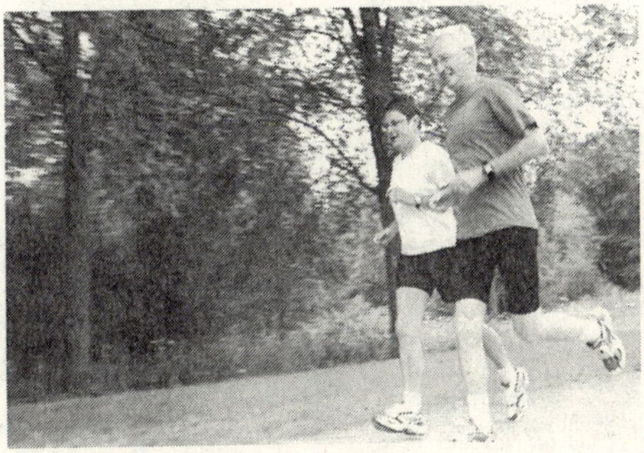

Calm Your Breathing to

When we examine the phenomenon of possession by evil spirits, we find that it usually takes place in parts of the body where the blood is congested and not flowing smoothly, or where exhaustion has set in. The back of the head is also a common target for possession, as are areas such as the neck, shoulders and hips, which are prone to stiffness.

So, people who are chronically in a state of possession and people who are easily possessed by evil spirits, such as those who return home completely exhausted after going out, whose bodies become heavy when they are among crowds, and whose necks and other joints begin to ache, should regulate the rhythm of the body.

You must focus on breathing, taking in fresh oxygen and visualizing your blood circulating slowly throughout your entire body, from your head, through your neck and shoulders, to your waist, and through all of your extremities without halt. When you do this, the discordant wavelengths will gradually move away from your body.

Remove Spiritual Influences

The best way to remove simple spiritual influences from your body is to begin by regulating the body itself. Extreme exhaustion is a sign of your blood thickening and clotting; carrying out light aerobic exercise will improve your blood's circulation, and will allow light to enter you more easily. Thereafter, you must gradually relax your body, regulate your breathing, and allow yourself to expand into a loose, free-flowing state of mind.

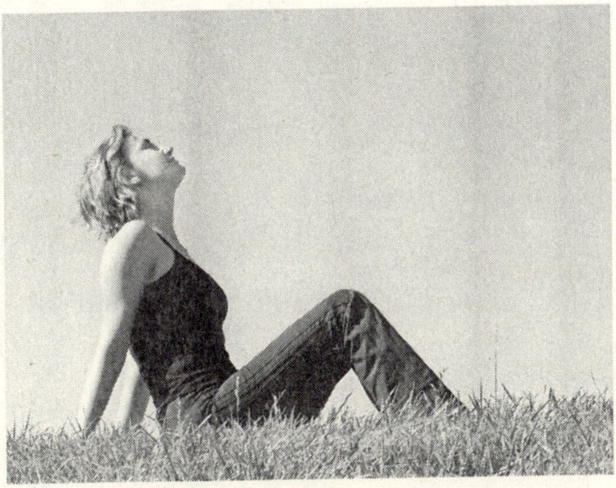

Part III

The Power of Faith is the Key to Good Health

Part III

The Power of Faith is the Key to Good Health

1

Your Body Reflects Your Own Self-Image

We human beings weigh a mere 3,000 grams or so when we are born; as we grow and age over the course of several decades, though, absolutely no part of our physical selves remain from the body that our parents gave to us when we came out of the womb.

The true nature of the physical body is like a flowing stream; every cell in our bodies is replaced. Our bone matter is changed out—even our skulls are renewed with the passing of time. The organs we have within us now are completely different from what we originally had. Not only are we not the same now as when we were born—we are still in the process of changing. Your body today is not the same as your body last month. A great portion of it is different. The body you had a year ago has been almost completely traded in for a new one. Every day, old cells are dying off and new cells are taking their place. This is the reality.

You may feel like saying, "I was born with a weak body," or, "It's all in the genes." However, if your body is still in the same poor condition as when you were born, it only means that you have continuously reproduced the same body. So how is it that you are able to maintain the same form even if your body is constantly changing?

The fact is that you have, within your own mind, a conception of who you are which is the blueprint your body follows. Your self image is producing your body. If you have ill will or a negative mind and are constantly telling yourself that you are sick and unhappy, sure to die soon, and can only live as a parasite upon the sympathy of others, then these thoughts will become a reality.

Within the body, there is an astral body, a spiritual body that is very close to the material world. Within this astral body, there are a great bundle of spiritual bodies that exist in a manifold structure. The signals that you transmit from your own mind are picked up by this astral body. Thus, whenever an abnormality takes place within the astral body, this abnormality appears in the physical body, as well. This is the root cause of diseases. Almost all illnesses are caused by our own minds.

This works in both directions, though. There is also a vicious circle in which the physical body is wounded, which hurts the astral body, which then influences the spiritual body. In Buddhism it is said, "The mind and matter are one." In other words, our physical bodies are in perfect accord with our minds. This is the way we are put together.

Ultimately, the star of the show is the mind; when the main character thinks to create a certain image, the astral body follows suit, and depending upon the degree of health of that body, different illnesses appear on the physical body.

When looked at in this way, every one of you has

Part III

The Power of Faith is the Key to Good Health

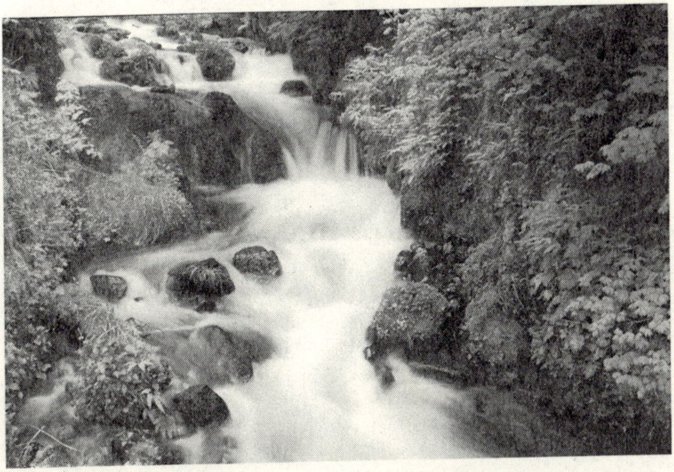

been given an enormous amount of possibility. You may be sick now, you may be sick in the future, or you might have been sick for a long time, but you must come to the realization that the body you have now is not the same body that you received from your parents when you were born.

2
Your Mind Determines Your Health

The subconscious mind exerts a great amount of influence upon both sickness and health. Some bodily activities are controlled by conscious thought, such as when you think about raising your arm, it moves exactly as you want it to. However, the vast majority of bodily functions are carried out subconsciously.

Would you be able to cause your blood to circulate by thinking about it? No, of course not. Nor could you coordinate your heart's beating through any form of conscious thought. Breathing, too, is an automatic process. While you are able to regulate your breathing, and while you have the power to consciously decide when and whether to breathe, under normal circumstances the body breathes on its own. Thus, many of the various body parts and cells operate in a realm outside of your consciousness. The subconscious controls most of the regions of your bodies.

Although many of you are surprisingly unaware of this fact, the regions of the body which are controlled by the subconscious have much more of an effect on your sickness and health than do the regions which you are free to move about as you wish, according to your conscious thoughts.

The human body has a multitude of cells, like the number of stars in the sky. From the point of view of

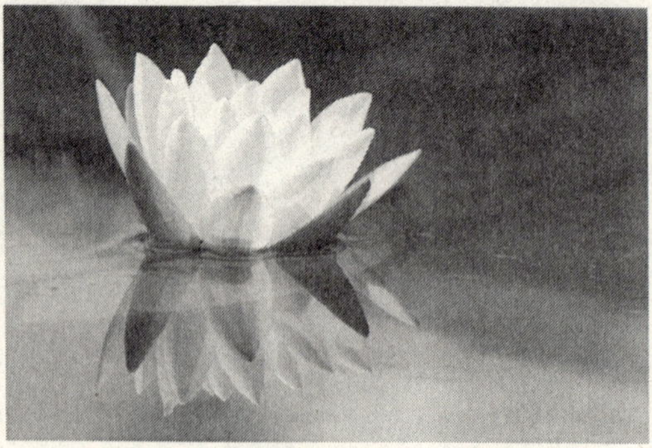

one of those cells, or of another microorganism living within the body, an internal organ is as vast as the galaxy. The swarm of living things within a human body is a confederation of separate life.

The power to create disease is also working in the realm of our subconscious. If, for example, we have negative thoughts within our surface consciousness, these ideas will sink deeply, like sediment, down into the depths of our subconscious. Then, they will become thought clouds of disease.

When these ideas of disease become present in the physical body, they are manifested as cancer and other disorders of the body's array of organs and tissues. There is a host of different diseases. Sickness attacks the liver, heart, lungs, kidneys, blood vessels, the brain, and so forth, but most of these sicknesses are the products of bad thoughts emitted over the decades, which have sunk deeply into our subconscious.

The subconscious has the power to make the physical body. When this power is misapplied, it can work towards destroying the self. Failure to understand this point can result in falling prey to disease.

The process outlined above usually causes cancer. Because cancer is a state in which the body is harboring cells which are actively seeking to destroy the body, it stands to reason that cancer must be caused by the patient having some sort of self-destructive bent of thought lodged deep within the mind. Moreover, in most cases, this comes about because of hatred or fear.

If you have been cruelly mistreated or horribly discriminated against in the past, then there is a good chance that you have bottled up a great deal of emotions such as hatred and anger within your heart. When these kinds of emotions accumulate, they become thought clouds of disease, eventually breeding cells within the body whose mission is to destroy the body.

However, if you have the power to create destructive cells, then you must also have the power to cure sickness. In other words, if you focus on thoughts that are the opposite of destructiveness, then the power to heal illnesses will begin to work.

3
The Power of Faith to Fight Cancer

People who develop cancer have harbored mistaken thoughts and led wayward lives for decades. These people have minds filled with hatred, anger, envy, jealousy, grudges, harsh words, and other such aggressive thoughts, which seek to ruin everything around them. These thoughts must be cleansed. You must reflect or seek the guidance of someone advanced in their enlightenment, and remove the ill thoughts that have accumulated in your mind.

A movie called *Spirited Away* came out several years back. This movie's director has an affinity with the minor realm of the spirit world, the world of mysterious creatures. In the movie, there is a scene in which there appears a smelly River God, whose entire body is filled with a gooey slime, which the heroine washes away with warm water.

People, whose thoughts are black through and through, are also covered in sludge like the River God in the movie. There are many of these kinds of people. If you live in such a state as this, it would actually be quite remarkable if you did not come down with any kind of disease, or experience some kind of accident, which affected either you or a member of your family. You must rinse yourself and be clear of negative thoughts like this slime.

Diseases can be cured by participating in ritual prayers at temples and local temples of Happy Science, but the truth is that you already possess the power to heal yourself. Everything will be set right again if you are able to teach a sick person the correct "Laws of the Mind," put them back on the right path, and turn them towards brightness and the heavenly world.

Medical science has recently learned that a great number of different kinds of sicknesses are ultimately caused by problems with the immune system. In fact, while you do possess the power to cure yourself of disease, when your immune functions are weakened, unwelcome things can enter your body and you can become sick and die.

However, immunity can actually be boosted through the power of belief and faith. This can also be attributed to the power of thoughts that come from the will of the individual in question, but when you live every day in the hopes to make effort as a bodhisattva for the sake of God, then your entire body becomes filled with a powerfully positive surge of good thoughts. Eventually they soak deep into all of your body's cells and work to raise your immunity.

When this occurs, then something like initial-stage cancer can be easily cured. Boosting your immunity can allow you to win your fight against cancer. It is also possible to pass this power of faith on to others. When you lead others with strong enthusiasm and set them on the right path, then their hearts will suddenly be filled with light, and their immune systems will be strengthened. Not only that, but every cell in their bodies will be given an increased power to live.

If you believe that you must keep pressing on, that you must do much more good work, then this will be transmitted to your cells, and your entire body will become more powerful. If you feel that you have a mission to fulfill, you will find that youthfulness will well up from within you, making you feel ten or twenty years younger.

4

Don't Fall in Love with Your Disease

While some diseases cannot be avoided, there are also many instances where someone's thoughts or mental states have welcomed the disease from which they presently suffer.

A sick person will not be very happy to hear that they are ill because they like being ill, but that is the truth in a great number of cases. There are many, many people who have failed in relationships with others or failed in their jobs, and who thus find themselves with no other escape than the asylum of disease. They believe that if they fall ill, all will be forgiven. They want to think that their sins have been dispelled by their sickness and that they are not responsible for their failures, and thus

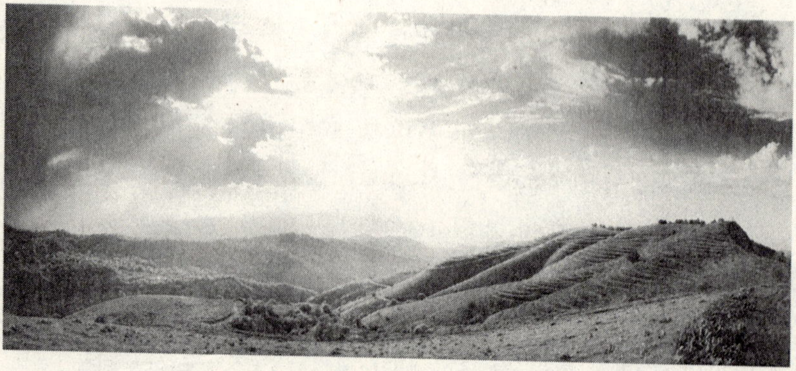

make themselves sick.

Even if they do not consciously think of this, these ideas are nevertheless present within their subconscious minds. They wish to fall ill, so they adopt unhealthy lifestyles, and begin doing things that they should not do, pushing themselves to the limit until they collapse and fall ill. These people then come to believe that they have been unlucky, and that fate has not been kind to them.

Illness furthermore has the added benefit of bringing sympathy to the afflicted. You must be aware, though, that some people have this tendency to wish to become ill, to want to escape through the medium of disease. It is a very prevalent state of mind.

How is it, then people whose minds are focused on success?

People who truly aim to succeed will recognize the early signs of illnesses and will consider taking good care of their body. They will seek out the advice of family and friends, and will eventually come to realize that they must change their working habits, for example, or whatever it might be that is ruining their health, after which they will take steps to make the appropriate adjustments.

Those who are in love with disease, though, will not listen to anyone's advice, however often it might be offered. They are told months before that if they keep up the current pace they would pay for it, but they do not listen and plow ahead, and then collapse. This is an example of irresponsibility being the cause of a disease.

Someone who truly feels a sense of responsibility will realize that if he becomes ill, it will cause many problems not only for him but for others as well. He will thus work to prevent health issues before they come to a head. Irresponsible people, though, disregard these warning signs, and end up placing a great burden upon everyone else as a result.

The entire question hinges upon whether, in your heart, you have an image of your own happiness, or a desire to live in unhappiness and failure.

Part III

The Power of Faith is the Key to Good Health

5

Recharge with the Power of Prayer

Some prayers are designed to replenish you with energy. When making such prayers, you must sit quietly and ask God to grant you infinite energy, unlimited wisdom, and boundless love.

While you are praying, visualize that wonderful energy is being supplied from Heaven, and that you are receiving this energy. Think, for example, that the infinite love of God is presently flowing into you. Then, when you feel that boundless love has filled your entire body, next turn your thoughts to how best to send this love out to everyone and everything in the world around you.

Repeat to yourself, "The infinite love of God is

flowing into me. I am receiving God's boundless strength." When you feel fully recharged, it is important to ask yourself how you can contribute this infinite power to the rest of the world.

I also engage in this practice. Some days I am worn out from my work and do not feel well. When I feel this way, I always ask for light from the high spirits. While I can also take in light from the heavenly world, I usually call on one of the high spirits and have them recharge me. The light simmers in and fills me with overflowing strength, and lets me tackle the next job I must do.

These requests are readily granted; many of the high spirits feel comfortable answering this request for light. The important thing is to be of a mindset wherein you take the light that you receive and then go out and use it to help everyone else around you.

Part III

The Power of Faith is the Key to Good Health

6

Prayer for Healing Illnesses —"El Cantare Healing"

According to His own Will, God created the universe, the sun, the stars, the flora, fauna of the Earth, and first among them, man. If God could do all of this on His own—if He could shine forth His light and make every whim a reality—then how could anyone think that He would be unable to flush out a trifling cluster of diseased cells inside of a human body?

Disease is a product of the mind, of a disharmony between the human mind and the body surrounding it. God can erase what a human has created. God is omnipotent. There is nothing, absolutely nothing that is impossible for Him, or that is beyond His reach.

God does not act because He has temporarily

entrusted all to human hands, but God possesses the power to erase this planet in the blink of an eye, and to create it just as quickly. This is the power of God. If you believe in this power, then all your diseases cannot continue to exist.

In Happy Science, there is a ritual prayer called, "El Cantare Healing," for healing diseases (practiced in the "Prayer for Recovery from Illnesses" in "Prayer Book 1," limited to Happy Science members). The prerequisite for this ritual prayer is that those who recite it have faith. If you do not have faith, then the light will not flow. If you do believe, though, then you will become one with the soul of El Cantare, and the light of healing will begin to come into you.

One way of performing this ritual prayer is to practice it directly in front of the person who is sick. Distance healing is another option. The particular feature of this method is that it is possible to heal someone who is away from you physically. In other words, the recipient of the prayer does not need to be in the same room in order to receive the healing benefits that the ritual prayer provides. The effectiveness of the prayer does not change even over hundreds of kilometers, even if you and the object of your prayer are on opposite sides of the globe.

If the person practicing the ritual prayer believes from the bottom of his heart that God has the power to freely make the Earth vanish as well as make it appear, then even cancerous cells will be erased. The important thing is to believe.

The New Testament tells us that Jesus was able to raise people from the dead. When Jesus came to the tomb of Lazarus and said, "Lazarus, come out!" Lazarus, wrapped in linen, arose from the slab and came out of the tomb, alive.

These events really happened in history. The reason why we cannot recreate this today is because humans have lost their power to believe. Even Christians have lost faith in the miracles that occurred in the time of Jesus.

Jesus brought dead men back to life. He made the blind to see, and made the physically disabled to walk again. He transformed water into wine. He multiplied loaves and fishes, and then fed a crowd of thousands. All of this was real, and true. Jesus turned these remarkable ideas into realities. The ones who choose to interpret these events as mere parables or metaphors are the modern Christians and Christian theologians. This is because these men and women do not know what a miracle is. They do not believe in the true power of God. Believe, and all things will be realized.

7
Faith Solves All Problems

Almost all modern diseases are caused by three factors—what we eat, lack of exercise, and stress. I think we can safely say that nearly every sickness is built upon these three unhealthy behaviors.

It is especially important that you begin taking steps in your mid-thirties to avoid developing what are known as "lifestyle diseases." Please take care of yourself, not only for your own sake and for the sake of your future, but also for the sake of your family. Do not be too easy on yourself and allow yourself to get away with unhealthy actions.

Diseases with clear-cut causes are diseases that can be prevented. If you continue to gorge on salty and high-calorie foods while ignoring exercise, then it is only a matter of time before you get sick. Going to banquets and parties, drinking, carousing, and stuffing yourself to the gills on a regular basis will definitely bring you illnesses.

In order to go on working into the future and to protect your family, it is important to practice moderation. Make every effort to protect what you can with your own hands.

Getting enough exercise will also require commitment on your part. You must make time for it, and must accept the fact that exercise brings with it a certain degree of discomfort. People say that they are too busy, but that is usually just an excuse. The real problem is that they are too lazy to try something new, so please do whatever it takes to make time for exercise. You cannot be stuck like glue to your coworkers through morning, noon and night. You need time alone.

The modern world is obsessed with going to the doctor's office, but doctor's offices and hospitals are centers of "black thinking," so you must be careful about visiting a physician. Doctors have a tendency to examine a patient and then to give that patient the absolute worst prognosis the doctor can possibly imagine. Do not be doomed by their words. Doctors are just trying to save their own skins by leading you to believe that you have one foot in the grave—that way, if you really do get worse, then they can't be blamed for it. In addition, if you improve, then the credit will be given to the doctor. This is why doctors spout off such depressing scenarios to those who visit them for a check-up.

However, immoderation such as overindulging in food and drink and refusing to get any exercise are not the entire story of why we become ill—our state of mind covers more than half of the reasons why we fall sick, which is why there are so many diseases which can be healed through "management of the mind."

In this sense, no matter how much your doctor says that you will never recover, or that you will have to go on taking medicine until you die, you must not take it

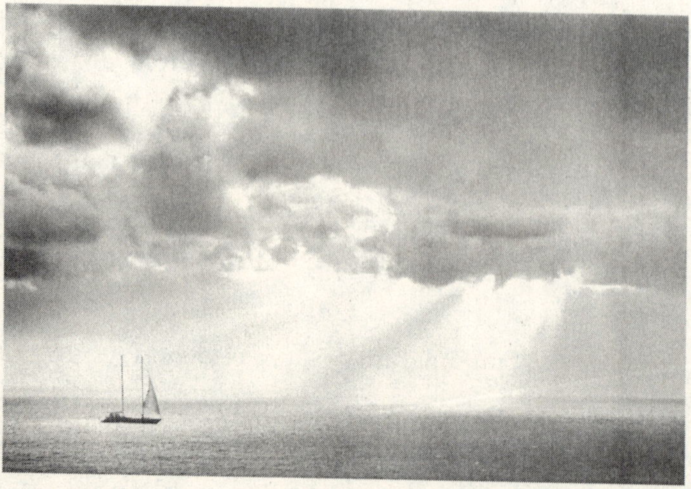

word for word. You must have the firm belief to resist this negative thinking, and to affirm that you are a child of God, and that you have the power to heal yourself. Tell yourself that you can heal your own body.

The body you have now is the total sum of all of the thoughts and emotions you have created. Whether it has been performed consciously or subconsciously, your body is the result of your own handiwork. If your body is sick, then it means that somewhere along the way you began to move in a negative direction; you must cultivate a strong desire to change, and then you must continue thinking that way. This is how change comes about.

Almost every disease is curable. Most illnesses including the top killers of Japanese people, such as cancer, heart disease, ailments of the brain and circulatory system, and others are originally supposed to be curable.

Of course, every human being is mortal, so death itself is inevitable. It is possible, though, to put death off until after you have passed through the most vibrant and important stages of your life. You have the power to avoid dying from illness, to go on living well, while you are doing important things at work, and while you are providing for your family.

Your faith and efforts are what will open the way forward for you. First, you must put forth all of the efforts that you are able to muster. If you smoke multipacks of cigarettes a day and then develop lung cancer as a result, God Himself will not be inclined to save you from the mess you have made. If you go through a bottle of whisky every night and end up ruining your liver, you should not expect any divine intervention. If you wish to heal your own body, then you must make an effort to change habits and behaviors that will clearly lead to disease at some point in the future.

You must undertake a complete reversal of the mind you have cultivated up until now, firmly understanding that things cannot continue as they have been, that disease must be cured, and that effort and faith are called for towards those ends.

Healing light and healing power can be found in the heavenly world. This light pours freely down onto those who believe and who make honest efforts to move forward. To tell the truth, the principle is the same as a teacher showing favoritism to some of the students. If a teacher thinks the children are adorable, then it stands to reason that that the children will receive more help from the teacher when needed.

Thus, it is incumbent upon you to become an "adorable child" in the eyes of God. You must live your life in a way that will be pleasing to God, and will cause Him to love you. Moreover, the most important thing in this regard is to have a right mind and to continue making daily efforts. In other words, you must be humble, you must love others, and you must be kind.

If you were to look inside the hearts of those who had fallen ill, you would almost invariably find them filled with hatred and anger. If you are sick, then reflect on your own mind. Is there anybody against whom you hold a grudge? If so, then the most important thing is to make peace with them. The hatred you feel towards

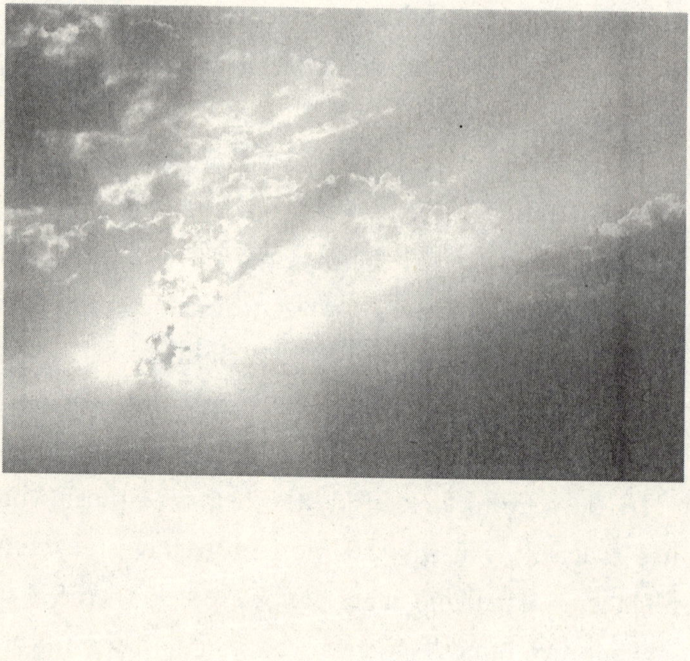

someone is what is bringing the illness to you, so you must stop hating whomever it is that you hate.

You may be placing all of the blame for something on someone else's shoulders, but I would wager that you have never tried to see things from the other person's standpoint, or from the point of view of God. The one-sided blame that you assign to other people, insisting that they are entirely in the wrong, that they have tortured you and that you therefore hate them for it, is only making you sick. It is not worth it.

It really is a foolish equation, isn't it? Would anyone really go out of his or her way to drink poison like that? No one is so foolish as to take poison while knowing that it would only make him or her sick. Hatred and anger, though, are exactly that—poisons.

Holding onto a grudge means, you are continuously destroying your own body. This hatred will surface as cancer or any other of a host of diseases. Holding a grudge is detrimental to you. If hatred is the cause of your sickness, then your sickness can be cured. First, you must reflect, and then your sickness will begin to improve.

If God looks upon you as one of His "adorable pupils," then He will feel inclined to grant you longer life. In fact, there are meetings in the heavenly world where it is decided whether to extend the span of someone's life or not. On most occasions, people get what they deserve, and there is nothing to be done about it. However, if decision is made in the heavenly world to grant someone longer life, then that particular person will live to witness the accumulation of their years.

All humans are mortal, though, so the high spirits will make a decision to allow someone to live only so long as they are needed on Earth. If the spirits of the heavenly world decree that, someone should be allowed to live, in almost all cases that person's diseases will be cured.

However, a person is responsible for more than ninety percent of all one's diseases. Almost every disease is just retribution for personal decisions, which is why it is difficult to completely overturn the results.

In addition, since the law of inertia is in force for the tendencies that you have built up over the decades of your life thus far, it is difficult to suddenly correct the course of your life. Religion, though, goes beyond secular logic, and has the power to resurrect us from our defeats and change us completely. Religion has the power to fundamentally change us. Not only can it cure diseases, it also has the strength to change the entire person. Thus, you should never give up hope. Regardless of how difficult your circumstances, you still have the chance to change.

There is a way through everything. When one door closes, another one always opens. Faith truly has the power to solve every problem you encounter. Nevertheless, faith requires effort on your part. Never forget the importance of effort and belief.

Modern Medicine and Religion

How should we understand the relationship
Between modern medicine and religion?
This is a challenging issue.

I do believe that modern medicine
Is guided by the divine spirits.
Here, let us call the angels of light in the field of medicine,
"Gods of Medicine."
When you trace the roots of the gods of Medicine,
You will eventually discover the god Hermes.

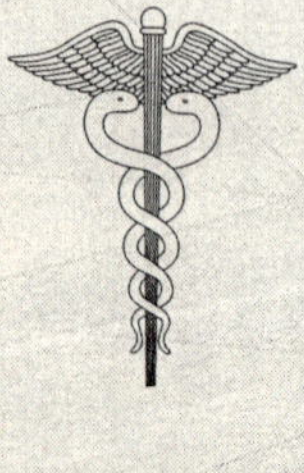

* God Hermes: A hero who lived in Greece 4,300 years ago. He brought prosperity to the Mediterranean area and laid the foundations of Western civilization. Well-known as the god of commerce, prosperity, the arts, travel and communications, among other things, Hermes is also a God of Healing. The Staff of Kerykeion (also known as the Caduceus Staff), which Hermes is often seen holding, is used even today as a symbol of medical institutions worldwide.

Eastern medicine
Sometimes conflicts with western medicine,
Having originated in the classic philosophies of
Lao-tzu and Chuang-tzu, and Buddhism.
There are actually many past examples
In which monks taught medicine.

The divine spirits are also providing ample guidance
To religions that heal people's illnesses.
From time to time, the divine spirits perform miracles
To deepen people's faith.

So, what is important is

The cooperation and collaboration

Between medicine and religion.

Physicians with religious faith

Should be able to heal more illnesses

By effectively using the power of the mind.

They should be able to miraculously cure

Even the most deadly illnesses

By combining positive words and medicine.

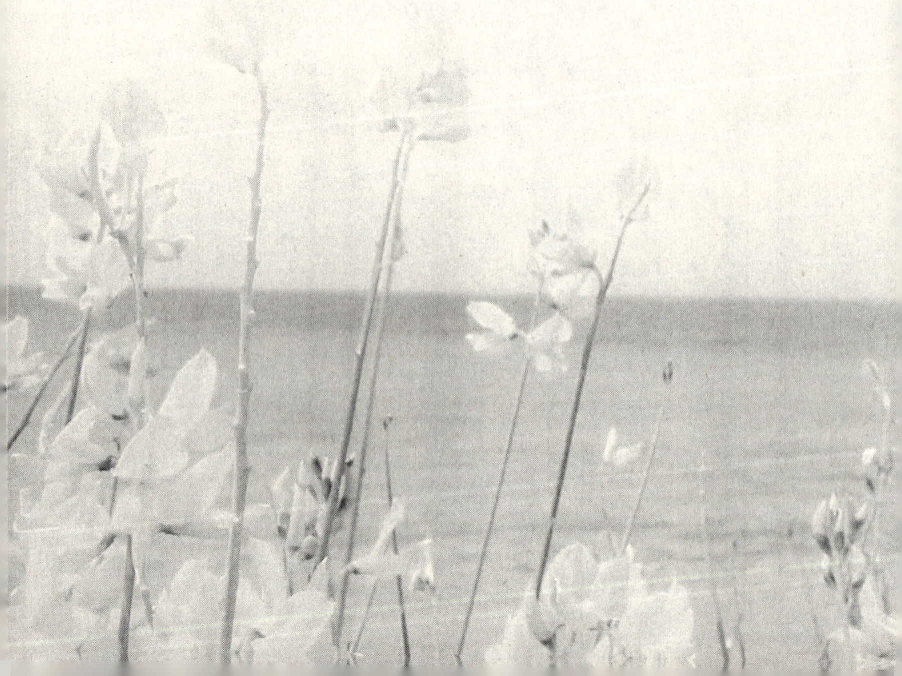

Likewise, people of religion should be capable
Of expanding the number of souls they save
By cooperating with the positive side of medicine.
The goal is people's happiness;
Therefore, cooperation is ideal.

Ryuho Okawa
President of Happy Science

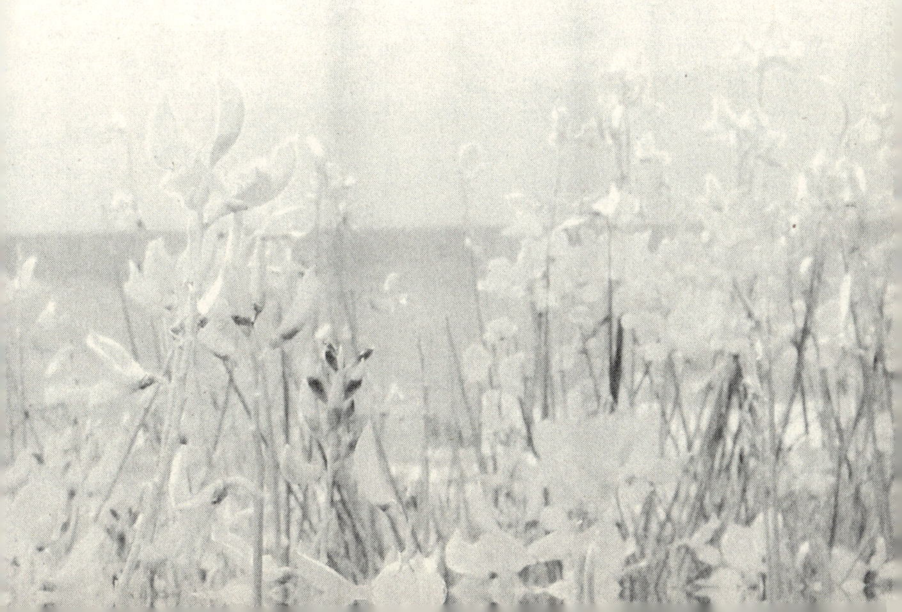

About the Author

Master Ryuho Okawa, founder of Happy Science and a world spiritual leader, has devoted much of his life to the exploration of the Truth and finding ways to bring True Happiness to people all over the world. He has given more than 1,800 lectures, and Happy Science under his guidance is a growing spiritual movement for the happiness of humanity since its founding in 1986. After graduating from the University of Tokyo, he joined a Tokyo-based trading house. While working at its New York headquarters, he studied finance at the Graduate Centre of the City University of New York. In 1986, he renounced his business career to establish Happy Science, which now has 12 million members in more than 90 countries. Master Okawa is also the author of more than 1000 books; in 2010, he published 52 books, setting the Guinness World Record for "most books written in one year by an individual." In Japan, Master Okawa's new books, published every year, have landed on the bestselling list for 21 consecutive years. His books have been translated into 25 languages.

Contact Information

Happy Science is a worldwide organization with faith centers around the globe. For a comprehensive list of centers, visit the Worldwide Directory at
happy-science.org
happyscience-na.org
ryuho-okawa.com
okawabooks.com

The following are a few of the many Happy Science locations:

International Headquarters:

Tokyo
1-6-7 Togoshi, Shinagawa,
Tokyo 142-0041, Japan
Tel: 81-3-6384-5770
Fax: 81-3-6384-5776
Email: tokyo@happy-science.org
Website: www.happy-science.org

India:

Delhi
Email: newdelhi@happy-science.org
Tel: 91-84476-88177

Mumbai
Email: mumbai@happy-science.org
Tel: 91-98192-64400

Aurangabad
Email: aurangabad@happy-science.org
Tel: 91-89561-01911

Tamil Nadu
tamilnadu@happy-science.org
Tel: 91-75069-72302

Kolkata
kolkata@happy-science.org
Tel: 91-70440-91597

Bodh Gaya
bodhgaya@happy-science.org
Tel: 91-82928-24767

Sri Lanka:

Colombo
Ground Floor No. 255, Dr. N.M. Parera Mawatha
Colombo 08
Email: srilanka@happy-science.org
Tel: 94-71-1544536

Nepal:

Sitapaila-15 Kimdol, Ward No. 15,
Kathmandu, Nepal
Email: nepal@happy-science.org
Tel: 977-14272-931

Join Happy Science

Anyone who wishes to study and follow Master Ryuho Okawa's teachings can join Happy Science as a member. The aim is to be truly happy and to share that happiness with others.

By becoming a member, you will receive a prayer book and periodical e-news letters which include the latest teachings of Master Ryuho Okawa. The prayer book contains three powerful prayers. By reciting these prayers each day you can cultivate your divine nature, receive inspiration and be spiritually protected.

Please send your email to the local branch email address as shown above, and they will get back to you shortly.

For your reference to Master Ryuho Okawa and Happy Science, you can browse the following website: http://www.happy-science.org/

Anyone who wishes to study Master Ryuho Okawa's teachings can sign up today to receive e-news letter in English or Hindi through the website: http://words.happyscience.me/

JAICO PUBLISHING HOUSE

Elevate Your Life. Transform Your World.

ESTABLISHED IN 1946, Jaico Publishing House is home to world-transforming authors such as Robin Sharma, Sadhguru, Osho, the Dalai Lama, Deepak Chopra, Eknath Easwaran, Paramhansa Yogananda, Devdutt Pattanaik, Radhakrishnan Pillai, Morgan Housel, Napoleon Hill, John Maxwell, Brian Tracy, and Stephen Hawking.

Our late founder Mr. Jaman Shah first established Jaico as a book distribution company. Sensing that independence was around the corner, he aptly named his company Jaico ('Jai' means victory in Hindi). In order to service the significant demand for affordable books in a developing nation, Mr. Shah initiated Jaico's own publications. Jaico was India's first publisher of paperback books in the English language.

While self-help; religion and philosophy; mind, body and spirit; and business titles form the cornerstone of our non-fiction list, we publish an exciting range of current affairs, history, biography, art and architecture, travel, and popular science books as well. Our renewed focus on popular fiction is evident in our new titles by a host of fresh young talent from India and abroad.

Jaico's translations division publishes select bestselling titles in over 10 regional languages including Gujarati, Hindi, Kannada, Malayalam, Marathi, Tamil, and Telugu. These include titles from renowned national and international authors like Sudha Murthy, Gaur Gopal Das, Swami Mukundananda, Jay Shetty, Simon Sinek, Ankur Warikoo and Jeff Keller.

Visit our Website

Boasting one of India's largest book distribution networks, Jaico has its headquarters in Mumbai, with branches in Ahmedabad, Bangalore, Chennai, Delhi, Hyderabad, and Kolkata. This network ensures that our books reach all parts of the country, both urban and rural.